Explaining Bi-Polar Disorder

Doreen Jarratt

Editor: Roger Sproston

Emerald Guides
www.straightforwardbooks.co.uk

Emerald Guides

© Straightforward Co Ltd 2024

All rights reserved. No part of this publication may be reproduced in a retrieval system or transmitted by any means, electronic or mechanical, photocopying or otherwise, without the prior permission of the copyright holder.

British Cataloguing in Publication Data. A catalogue record is available for this book from the British library.

ISBN

978-1-80236-318-0

Printed by 4edge www.4edge.co.uk

Cover design by BW Studio Derby

Whilst every effort has been taken to ensure that the information in this book is accurate at the time of going to press, the author and publisher recognise that the information can become out of date. This is particularly relevant to legal information. The book is therefore sold on the understanding that no responsibility for errors and omissions is assumed and no responsibility is held for the information held within.

Contents

Ch 1. Introduction 5

Ch 2 Bi-polar Disorder-Support and Self-help-Taking Control of Your Situation 19

Ch 3. Treatment for Bi-polar Disorder-Medication 29

Ch 4. Professional Help and Support 40

Ch 5. More about behavioural therapies 51

Ch 6. Dealing With Stigma and Shame 58

Ch 7. Bipolar Disorder and Vicious Cycles 64

Ch 8. Assertiveness-the Importance of Being Assertive 74

Ch 9. The Risks of Sleep Loss 79

Ch 10. Bipolar Disorder-Family Issues 86

Ch 11. Bipolar disorder and diet 92

Ch 12. Rights in the workplace 100

Chapter 13. Welfare Benefits and Bipolar Disorder   110

Conclusion

Useful addresses and websites

Index

Appendix 1-A Comprehensive outline of Welfare Benefits and other help available for bi-polar sufferers.

****

Chapter 1

Introduction

This book is intended to provide a comprehensive overview of the condition known as bipolar disorder. The book, updated to 2024, and written in recognition of World Bi-Polar day in March 2024, aims to be of use to those who have the condition and also family and friends who are affected by the condition.

This book is not an academic text but aims to be informative for those who want to know more about the condition. For more up to date current research and findings go to: www.bipolaruk.org.

What is bipolar disorder?
Bipolar disorder is the term used to describe what was once known as manic depression. Bipolar disorder causes serious shifts in mood, energy, thinking and behaviour. Essentially, if you have bipolar disorder, you will experience extreme swings in mood-from periods of hyperactivity, known as 'mania' or 'manic episodes' to deep depression. Some people also see or hear things around them that others don't (known as visual or auditory hallucinations) or have uncommon, unshared beliefs (known as delusions). In periods of calm, usually through some

form of medication, you will find yourself 'level' and behaving normally.

Signs and symptoms of bi-polar disorder There are four types of mood episode in bipolar disorder: mania, hypomania, depression and mixed episodes.

Manic episodes

In the manic phase of bipolar disorder, feelings of heightened energy, creativity, and euphoria are common. People experiencing a manic episode often talk very fast, sleep very little and are hyperactive Such a person may feel that they are all-powerful, invincible, or destined for greatness. To summarise, symptoms might include:

- A feeling of euphoria
- Feelings of restlessness
- Extreme irritability
- Talking very fast
- Racing thoughts
- lack of concentration
- Lots of energy
- A reduced need for sleep
- A sense of own importance
- Poor judgement
- Excessive and inappropriate spending

- Increased sexual drive
- Risky behaviour
- Misuse of drugs or alcohol
- Aggressive behaviour.

While mania might feel good in the first instance, it tends to spiral out of control. The aggressive side of mania can be a particular problem, picking fights, lashing out and so on.

Hypomania

Hypomania is a less severe form of mania. people in a hypomanic state feel euphoric, energetic and productive, but they are able to carry on with their day-to-day lives and they never lose touch with reality. To others, it may seem that people with hypomania are in an unusually good mood. However, hypomania can result in bad decisions that can harm relationships with others and also harm careers and reputations. In addition, hypomania can also escalate to a full-blown mania.

Depression

In the past, bipolar depression was seen as general depression. Doctors couldn't differentiate. However, a growing body of research suggests that there is a significant difference between the two, especially when it comes to recommended treatments. Whereas doctors tend to prescribe anti-depressants in many cases, these will not always help those with bipolar disorder. In fact, it has been proved that they can make the condition worse, triggering mania.

Despite many similarities, certain symptoms are more common in bipolar depression than in regular depression. For example, bipolar depression is more likely to involve irritability, guilt, unpredictable mood swings and restlessness. People with bipolar depression also tend to move and speak slowly, sleep a lot and gain weight. In addition, they are more likely to develop psychotic depression-a condition where a person loses contact with reality and also to experience major problems with social functioning, which can affect work. Common symptoms of bipolar depression include:

- Feeling hopeless, sad or empty
- Irritability
- Inability to experience pleasure
- Fatigue or loss of energy
- Physical or mental sluggishness
- Appetite or weight changes
- Sleep problems
- Concentration and memory problems
- Feelings of worthlessness or guilt
- Thoughts of death or suicide.

Signs and symptoms of a mixed episode

A mixed episode of bipolar disorder, as its name suggests, is where a person will exhibit symptoms of mania, hypomania and depression. Common signs of a mixed episode include depression combined with agitation, irritability, anxiety, distractibility and racing thoughts. This combination of moods makes for a very high risk of suicide.

Different types of bipolar disorder
Bipolar disorder is further categorized as:
-Bipolar 1 disorder, which is mania or mixed episode. This is the classic manic-depressive form of the illness, characterized by at least one manic or mixed episode. Usually, but not in all cases, bipolar 1 will involve at least one episode of depression.

-Bipolar 2 disorder (hypomania and depression). In bipolar 2 disorder the person doesn't experience full blown manic episodes. Instead, the illness involves a mixture of hypomania and severe depression.

-Cyclothymia (hypermania and mild depression). Cyclothymia is a milder form of bipolar disorder. It consists of cyclical mood swings. However, the symptoms are less severe than full-blown mania or depression.

Length and frequency of episodes
A person may have very few bipolar disorder episodes, with years of stability in between each episode. However, they may also experience many more. Episodes can vary in length and

frequency from weeks to months, with varying lengths of time in between.

Mania usually starts suddenly and lasts between two weeks and four to five months. Depression often lasts longer, on average around six months, but can last longer, but usually less than a year.

Although a person may cope very well in between episodes, they may experience low-level symptoms in these relatively 'stable' periods which can impact on daily life.

What causes bipolar disorder?
Like a lot of other conditions, for example, Parkinson's, very little is known about the sources of bipolar disorder. However, it does run in families, which suggests a genetic link. On the other hand, there may not be a family link and the origin may lie elsewhere. This is one of the problems with diagnosing the causes of bipolar disorder. Unless the link is obvious then the origins remain obscure. The disorder is diagnosed in a roughly equal number of men or women. It usually starts in the 20's and 30's, although it can also start as a teenager.

The fact that symptoms can be controlled by medication, especially lithium and anticonvulsants (see chapter 3) suggests that there may be problems with the functions of the nerves in the brain. This is supported by research. Disturbances in the endocrine system (controlling hormones) may also be involved. Most research suggests that a stressful environment, social factors, or physical illness may trigger the condition. Although stress is unlikely to cause bipolar disorder, it seems to be a significant trigger. A person may find that the start of bipolar episodes can be linked to a period of great stress, such as childbirth, a relationship breakdown, money problems or a career change. Sleep disturbance can be an important contributor.

Childhood distress
Some experts believe that a person may develop bipolar disorder if they experienced severe emotional damage in early life, such as physical, sexual or emotional abuse. Grief, loss trauma and neglect can be contributory factors-they can shock the developing mind and produce unbearable stress.

General problems in life
It is also very possible that bipolar disorder can be a reaction to overwhelming problems in day-to-day life. Mania can be a way of escaping unbearable depression. For example, if a person appears to have very over-inflated sense of one's own self-importance and place in society, they may be compensating for a severe lack of self-confidence and lack of self-esteem.

Childhood bi-polar disorder
Childhood bipolar disorder, also known as pediatric bipolar disorder, is a form of bipolar disorder that occurs, as its name

suggests, in children. While its existence is still a matter of academic debate and disagreement, there is a growing body of evidence that suggests that bipolar disorder can exist in children.

Unlike most adults who have bipolar disorder, however, children who have pediatric bipolar disorder are characterized by abrupt mood swings, periods of hyperactivity followed by lethargy, intense temper tantrums, frustration and defiant behavior. This rapid and severe cycling between moods may produce a type of chronic irritability with few clear periods of peace between episodes.

Because the current diagnostic manual of mental disorders doesn't recognize childhood bipolar disorder, there is no official symptom criteria. However, researchers have used criteria similar to that of adult bipolar disorder, requiring a child or teen to meet at least four or more of the following:

- an expansive or irritable mood
- extreme sadness or lack of interest in play
- rapidly changing moods lasting a few hours to a few days
- explosive, lengthy, and often destructive rages
- separation anxiety
- defiance of authority
- hyperactivity, agitation, and distractibility
- sleeping little or, alternatively, sleeping too much
- bed-wetting and night terrors
- strong and frequent cravings, often for carbohydrates and sweets

- excessive involvement in multiple projects and activities
- impaired judgment, impulsivity, racing thoughts, and pressure to keep talking
- dare-devil behaviors (such as jumping out of moving cars or off roofs)
- inappropriate or precocious sexual behavior
- grandiose belief in own abilities that defy the laws of logic (ability to fly, for example).

Keep in mind that many of these behaviors, in and of themselves, are not indicative of a possible disorder and are characteristic of normal childhood development. For instance, separation anxiety, by itself, is a normal fear of being separated from one or both of the parents (for instance, attending the first day of school or if the parents want to go out for a night).

Childhood bipolar disorder is characterized by many of these symptoms, taken together, and marked by rapid mood swings and hyperactivity. These symptoms must also cause significant distress in the child or teen, occur in more than just one setting (e.g. at school and at home), and last for at least 2 weeks.

Bi-Polar disorder-implications for pregnancy and childbirth

For any women (and man) having a baby is a major event and quite often a stressful time Women with bipolar disorder, and their families and friends, will have numerous questions to which they will need answers.

Common questions might be:
- Will the birth of the baby affect me in any way, will I become ill?
- Is bipolar hereditary-will my children develop bipolar disorder?
- Will my medication affect my pregnancy and my baby?

Firstly, each woman's experience is unique, therefore it is difficult to give general answers to questions that will apply to all women.

Discussing pregnancy with your GP and psychiatric team

It is best to discuss issues surrounding pregnancy before you even start to try for a baby. Some GP's and psychiatrists have a special interest in psychiatric illness and childbirth, which is sometimes called Perinatal psychiatry. Not all areas in the UK are covered by Perinatal teams. If you are fortunate enough to live in an area where there is a team, then you can be referred to them. If there is no local service then you may have to travel.

A few questions answered

1. Risks of becoming ill during pregnancy and after childbirth

Women with bipolar disorder may become unwell during pregnancy but are at a particularly high risk of becoming ill following childbirth. There is a risk of severe manic and depressive episodes. In addition, mood symptoms such as elation, irritability and depression can occur, along with psychotic symptoms such as delusions and hallucinations. When such symptoms are severe it may be called an episode pf postpartum psychosis or puerperal psychosis. Other mood episodes at this time may be labelled as 'postnatal depression' or 'postpartum depression'. Women who experience severe episodes following pregnancy may require hospitalisation but usually respond well to treatment.

Two groups of women with bipolar disorder are at higher risk: those who have had a previous period of severe illness following childbirth, and those with a relative who has suffered postpartum psychosis. Women with bipolar disorder must think very carefully about these risks before becoming pregnant.

2. What can I do to lower the risks of becoming ill?

The main thing here is to ensure that you let all those involved know that you have bipolar disorder and that there is a real risk of becoming unwell again after childbirth. Your midwife, GP, health visitor and obstetrician should all be made aware of your bipolar and of your past history. Anyone else who is involved with you such as your CPN or psychiatrist should also be told. As discussed above, you should inform everyone who is relevant before you become pregnant.

Paying attention to other issues known to increase the risk of becoming ill may be important. These include trying to reduce other stressful things going on in your life. paying attention to sleep, before and after your baby is born is important. With a new baby, this can be difficult but you will need as much support as possible from your partner.

3. Will my children contact bi-polar disorder?

It is a fact that many illnesses run in families. This is true for all sorts of conditions, such as diabetes, heart conditions and cancer, but also for psychiatric disorders. However, although the children of people with bipolar disorder may be at a higher risk of becoming ill than people in general it is by no means a foregone conclusion. Only about 10% of children who have a parent with illness develop it themselves, so the majority are likely to stay well.

4. Will my medication affect my pregnancy?

On the whole, most medications present a low risk. However, it is necessary to discuss this with your GP who will have a better idea of any side effects of a particular drug. One thing is certain, stopping medication suddenly can increase the risks of illness.

5. Will my condition affect breastfeeding?

Whilst it is possible to breastfeed while taking some medications, you need to be fully aware of the risks involved. It may be that you are unable to breastfeed. There are several reasons why this is the case. You may be too unwell or you may be admitted to hospital without your baby. You may need a medication which is not safe in breastfeeding. Additionally, getting up in the night to breastfeed may cause sleep deprivation, or exacerbate the sleep deprivation that you are already experiencing which poses a risk to you.

6. What sort of care will I receive during pregnancy?
If you have bipolar disorder, it is important that you receive specialist care during pregnancy. If Perinatal treatment is available in your area, you should see the team, if not you should see a psychiatrist. The outcome should be a written care plan for you. Your midwives will also offer support during this period.

When you go home after you have had your baby, your mental health should be closely monitored. Your midwife, health visitor and mental health nurse should visit regularly in the first few weeks after your baby is born. If you become unwell during this period this can be picked up quickly so you can get early treatment.

In the next chapter, we will look at what you can do to help yourself if you have been diagnosed with bipolar disorder. Having understood something about the nature of bipolar disorder by reading this chapter, it is now time to understand what you can do to ensure that you can at least have as normal a life as possible.

Now read the main points from chapter one overleaf.

Main points from Chapter One

- Bipolar disorder is the term used to describe what was once known as manic depression. Bipolar disorder causes serious shifts in mood, energy, thinking and behaviour.

- There are four types of mood episode in bipolar disorder: mania, hypomania, depression and mixed episodes.

- Like a lot of other conditions, for example, Parkinson's, very little is known about the sources of bipolar disorder. However, it does run in families, which suggests a genetic link. On the other hand, there may not be a family link and the origin may lie elsewhere.

- Childhood bipolar disorder, also known as pediatric bipolar disorder, is a form of bipolar disorder that occurs, as its name suggests, in children. While its existence is still a matter of some academic debate and disagreement, there is a growing body of evidence that suggests that bipolar disorder can exist in children.

- Bipolar disorder can affect women who are pregnant and also have implications after childbirth. It is highly advisable to consult your GP and mental health team about issues surrounding pregnancy.

Chapter 2

Bipolar Disorder-Support and Self-Help-Taking Control of Your Situation

---

In chapters 3 and 4, we will be looking at medication and other treatments available to help you control your condition. However, before we describe these there are some general tips that are essential to ensure that you stay in control of your day-to-day life and don't let bipolar disorder control you. Everything that we discuss here will be discussed in more depth as we progress through the book.

Living with bipolar disorder-what you can do to help yourself
If you want to live a decent life with bipolar disorder, and not let it control you, you need to control the condition. This principle applies to many conditions that affect the way people interact on a day-to-day basis. It is very important that you make right and healthy choices for yourself. Doing so will minimise mood episodes, or minimise the effects of these on you and others.

Managing bipolar disorder starts with proper treatment, including medication and therapy. However, there is so much more that you can do to help yourself on a day-to-day basis. The medical profession and other professions that have involvement with you can only go so far. The rest is up to you.

There are key recovery concepts that are fundamental to self-help in managing bipolar disorder:

- *Self-belief, faith in yourself and hope.* With effective symptom management it is very possible to experience prolonged periods of wellness. Believing that you can cope with your mood disorder is essential to future recovery. This is the main tenet, belief, hope and faith in yourself. I have known people who revert to drink out of a sense of hopelessness which is exactly the wrong thing to do. Don't revert to drink, revert to your own inner strength.
- *Taking responsibility.* This follows on from the first principle. It is up to you to take action to keep your moods stabilised. This includes asking help from others when needed, not keeping yourself buttoned up, too proud to open up. Take your medication as prescribed and keep appointments with health care providers.
- *Self- advocacy.* This means being assertive and ensuring that you get the best treatment and support for yourself. In the end, it is you as an individual that is affected and you must represent yourself. Open up to professionals and make sure that they are providing you with the best service.

- *Educate yourself.* Make sure that you understand everything about your condition. Only when you are enlightened can you make sure that you know what you want and how to get it.

Finally, support. Support from others is essential to maintain your stability and enhance your quality of life. Support means from family, friends and professionals.

Know your early warning signs

It is very important to know the warning signs of an oncoming manic or depressive episode. In order to recognize them, you should have a list of the previous symptoms that preceded earlier episodes. You should try to identify the triggers that have caused the onset of an episode in the past, what the influences were. If they were outside influences, then what were they? Common triggers can be:

- Stress-a very common trigger.
- Arguments with loved ones including family.
- Problems at school or work.
- Lack of sleep.
- Too much alcohol.

What you are trying to achieve here is a form of self-monitoring so you are building up an historical pattern which will aid you in the future. Get to know yourself and put yourself in a position where you can recognize episodes as they happen or are beginning to happen. One way of monitoring your symptoms is by keeping a mood chart. Although this might seem laborious, in fact it can provide valuable information about your emotional state and other symptoms that you are having. It can also include information such as how much sleep you are getting, what your sleep patterns are, your diet and alcohol intake and also your medication and how this is affecting you.

Putting together a personal self-help pack

Building on from the above, if you spot any early warning signs of mania or depression, it is important to act quickly, in order to stay in control. In such times, you need a *self-help pack* to draw from. This consists of actions that you can take at any one given time. Many people with bipolar disorder have found the following to be helpful in reducing symptoms and maintaining well-being:

- Talk to a supportive person
- Make sure you get a full eight hours sleep
- Cut back on activities
- Attend a support group
- Talk regularly (as possible) to your doctor or therapist
- Ensure that you take time to relax and unwind
- Keep regular notes, as discussed above
- Make sure that you exercise regularly

- Cut back on sugar, alcohol and caffeine
- Increase exposure to light.

Create an emergency action plan

As with everything in life, it is always best to have an action plan that you can refer to if you run into trouble. When your own safety is at stake you may have to act quickly. A plan of action should include:
- A list of emergency contacts (doctor, therapist, family members)
- A list of all medications that you are taking, including dosage information
- Information about any other health problems that you have
- Symptoms that indicate that you need others to take responsibility for your care
- Treatments preferences-i.e. a list of medications that do not work-who is authorised to take decisions on your behalf etc.

Having a strong support system is vital to staying happy and stable. Creating a supportive environment includes not only who you choose to surround yourself with but also who to avoid, such as people who drain your energy or leave you feeling negative. Spend time with people who value you and leave you feeling positive about yourself.

Develop a daily routine

Your lifestyle choices will have a significant impact on your moods. These choices include sleeping patterns, eating and exercise patterns and the other many things that you do in your daily life to keep depression at bay.

Build structure into your life. Developing and sticking to a daily schedule can help stabilize the mood swings of bipolar disorder. Include set times for sleeping, eating, socializing, working and relaxing. Try to maintain regular patterns of activity even through emotional ups and downs.

Exercise regularly. Exercise has a beneficial impact on mood and may reduce the number of bipolar episodes that you experience. Aerobic exercise is especially effective at treating depression. Try to incorporate at least 30 minutes of activity at least five times a week into your routine. Walking is also a good choice, for people of all fitness levels.

Keep a strict sleep schedule. Getting too little sleep can trigger mania. It is very important indeed to ensure that you get lots of rest. It is important to get the balance right between too little and too much sleep. The best advice here is to maintain a normal sleep schedule, going to bed at the same time every night and rising at the same time.

Stress

Keep stress to a minimum. Stress can trigger episodes of mania and depression in people with bipolar disorder. Know your limits in life and don't take on too much. Learn how to relax. Relaxation techniques such as deep breathing, yoga, meditation can help improve mood and keep depression at bay.

Make leisure time a priority. Do things for no other reason than it feels good to do them. Switch off, read a book, go away on holiday watch a film. Above all, make sure that this is uninterrupted time to yourself.

Diet and bipolar disorder
From the food you eat to any vitamins that you take, what you put into your body is of vital importance. This applies to everyone, not just those with bi-polar disorder. Eat a healthy diet. For optimal mood eat plenty of fruit and vegetables and whole grains, avoid excessive sugar and also fat intake. Space your meals throughout the day and ensure that your blood sugar doesn't get too low. High carbohydrates can cause mood crashes. Other damaging foods include chocolate, caffeine and processed foods.

Omega 3 fatty acids may decrease mood swings in bi-polar disorder. Omega 3 is available as a nutritional supplement. You can also increase your intake of omega 3 by eating cold-water fish such as salmon, sardines and halibut. Soya beans, pumpkin seeds and walnuts also have a high omega 3 content. We will be expanding on the importance of diet later in the book.

Avoid alcohol and drugs at all costs. Drugs such as marijuana, cocaine, ecstasy and tranquilizers can all trigger depression and affect moods. Even moderate social drinking can upset your balance.

Be cautious when taking medication. Certain prescription and over the counter medications can be problematic for people with bi-polar disorder. Be especially careful with anti-depressant drugs, which can trigger mania. Other drugs that can cause mania include over-the-counter cold medicine, appetite suppressants, caffeine, corticosteroids and thyroid medication.

In the next chapter, we will look at the nature of the different types of medication available to treat bipolar disorder.

.

Now read the main points from Chapter Two overleaf.

****

Main points from Chapter Two

- If you want to live a decent life with bi-polar disorder, and not let it control you, you need to control the condition. This principle applies to many conditions that affect the way people interact on a day-to-day basis. It is very important that you make right and healthy choices for yourself. Doing so will minimise mood episodes or minimise the effects of these on you and others.

- There are key recovery concepts that are fundamental to self-help in managing bi-polar disorder: *Self-belief, faith in your-self and hope, taking responsibility, self- advocacy, educating your-self* and finally, *support from professionals.*

- It is very important to know the warning signs of an oncoming manic or depressive episode. In order to recognize them, you should have a list of the previous symptoms that preceded earlier episodes. You should try to identify the triggers that have caused the episode in question.

- As with everything in life, it is always best to have an action plan that you can refer to if you run into trouble. When your own safety is at stake you may have to act quickly.

- From the food you eat to any vitamins that you take, what you put into your body is of vital importance. Eat a healthy diet. For optimal mood eat plenty of fruit and vegetables and whole grains, avoid excessive sugar and also fat intake. Space your meals throughout the day and ensure that your blood sugar doesn't get too low. High carbohydrates can cause mood crashes.

- Be cautious when taking medication.

****

Chapter 3

Treatment for Bipolar Disorder-Initial Diagnosis and Medication

If your GP thinks that you have bi-polar disorder, they may refer you to a psychiatrist. Your psychiatrist or GP should explain all of your options to you and your views should be taken into account before your treatment starts.

NICE Guidance
The National Institute for Health and Care Excellence (NICE) www.nice.org.uk has guidelines for the treatment of bipolar disorder. They suggest that you should be offered structured psychological treatment while you are relatively stable but may be experiencing mild to moderate symptoms.

Usually, the psychological treatment would be given in addition to medication and you should be offered at least 16 sessions. The treatment should cover:
- Education about the illness-including information about the importance of regular daily routine and sleep, and about any medication that you have agreed to take

- How to monitor your mood, detect early warning signs and strategies to prevent symptoms from developing into full-blown episodes
- General coping strategies.

Virtually everyone who has been diagnosed with bipolar disorder will receive medication of one sort or another. Although drugs cannot cure bipolar disorder they help to manage the symptoms. Drugs used include lithium, anticonvulsants and anti-psychotics. It is very important to ensure that you have a full understanding of the medication offered and that you monitor your physical health.

Learning about bi-polar disorder medication
When starting medication for bipolar disorder, you should make sure that you know how to take it safely. Questions that you should ask your doctor include:
- Are there any medical conditions that exacerbate my mood swings? For example, an overactive thyroid gland may mimic the symptoms of bipolar disorder. You should ask your GP to carry out a simple blood test to ascertain this.
- What are the side effects and risks of the medication that is being recommended?
- When and how should the medication be taken?

- Are there any foods or other substances that I should avoid?
- How will the medication interact with my other prescriptions?
- How long will I take this medication for?
- Will withdrawing from the drug be difficult once I start?
- Will my symptoms return once I start taking the medication?

These might seem basic questions and you might expect your GP to answer them as a matter of course. However, this doesn't always happen, so, as explained in the last chapter, make sure that you are in control.

During acute mania or depression, you should talk with your doctor at least once a week, or more frequently, to monitor symptoms. As time goes by and you stabilise then you will see your GP less frequently. Once again, it is up to you to see that this happens.

Types of medication
Lithium
Lithium is a mood stabilizer and is the most common form of medication for those with bipolar disorder. It is the most effective medication for treating mania. It can also help depression. However, it is not really effective for mixed

episodes. Lithium will take between one to two weeks to take effect.

Lithium is a naturally occurring element, the lightest of the metals and comes as two different salts: Lithium carbonate (Camcolit, Liskonum, Priadel) and Lithium Citrate (Li-Liquid, Priadel). It does not matter which of these that you take, but you should keep to the same one, because they are absorbed slightly differently.

It is very important that lithium is taken at the right level and regular blood tests are essential. It is also very important to drink plenty of fluids every day and alcohol should be taken in moderation as well as coffee and strong tea.

Common side effects of lithium

There are a number of side effects of lithium, both common side effects and more serious. The common side effects are increased thirsts and urination, dry mouth, trembling hands, mild nausea and acne. The more serious side effects are weight gain, excessive urination, thyroid and kidney damage. Toxic effects that can arise as a result of too much lithium in the blood are diarrhoea, intense thirst, persistent nausea and vomiting, confusion, severe tremors and blurred vision. If you are taking lithium and suffer any of these symptoms then it is very important that you have a blood test, as failing to do so can result in kidney damage.

Avoiding toxic lithium levels from developing

There are ways that you can exercise control over the amount of lithium in your blood:
- Make sure that you go for blood tests when they are needed
- Don't suddenly change the amount of salt in your diet
- Make sure that you drink enough fluids
- Control your alcohol intake-keep it to a bare minimum
- See a doctor straight away if you feel that you are developing symptoms relating to toxicity.

Anticonvulsant drugs

Some other drugs are commonly used as mood stabilizers, Sodium valproate and Carbamazepine plus Lamotrigine. Although both were initially used for the management of epilepsy, they have been found to offer benefits to bi-polar patients. Sodium valproate, (common names: Epilim, Divalproex, Depakote) has been found to be effective in patients who suffer predominantly from depression. Common side effects can be: Nausea, vomiting, weight gain, tremors, drowsiness, hair loss.

Carbamazepine, (common name: Tegretolks), works less well in such cases. Common side effects: Dry mouth, nausea, diarrhoea, dizziness, headaches, problems with walking, tiredness and rashes.

Lamotrigine has anti-depressant effects and is licensed for depressive episodes in bipolar disorder. Like lithium, anticonvulsants also have to be monitored for excess levels, although not as tightly as lithium. They can also present some risk during pregnancy

Anti-depressants

As we discussed earlier in chapter one, anti-depressants are not the most effective drugs for those with bipolar disorder. There are a number of different types of anti-depressants, but the two most commonly prescribed are the Trcyclic anti-depressants (TCA's) and the serotonin reuptake inhibitors (SSRI's). The first type has been in use a long time now and the second type for about ten years. Both are effective and both take between two weeks and a month to relieve depression. However, both types of drugs have differing side effects.

In bi-polar disorder, these drugs may be used during depressive episodes. However, as mentioned the side effects can present a danger. There is a risk, in some people that anti-depressants can trigger an episode of mania. People with bi-polar should probably be on a mood stabilizer if taking anti-depressants and, as a rule, not take them for more than six months.

The TCA's

Examples of these drugs include Amitriptyline (Lentizol/Elavil), dothiepin/dosulepin (prothiaden) and lofepramine (Gamanil).

Side effects of these drugs: they have a wide variety of side effects, which are often more pronounced during the early stages of taking the drug. Common side effects include tiredness and excessive sedation, dry mouth, constipation and difficulty in urinating. After the first few weeks, these side effects should decrease.

The SSRI's

Examples include fluoexetine (Prozac), paroxetine (Seroxat, paxil) citalopram (Cipramil, Cipram) and sertraline (Lustral, Zoloft). There are also some newer, related antidepressants, including venlafaxine (Efexor) and nefazodone (Dutonin). All of these drugs have weird and wonderful names, but some are more well know than others, such as Prozac, which has had a lot of bad press.

Side effects: these drugs are said to have fewer side effects than the trycyclics and are, supposedly, safer in the event of an overdose. However, they can have a number of varied side effects, including upset stomach, headaches, agitation and rashes. Like most side effects they subside over time. One other class of anti-depressant that is sometimes prescribed is the monoamine oxidase (MAO) inhibitors. These were the first antidepressants, but most of them cannot be mixed with certain foods, such as cheeses and yeast products. For this reason, they are rarely prescribed. However, a new type of MAO inhibitor, moclobemide (Manerix) does not require dietary restriction.

Antipsychotic drugs (Neuroleptics)

Some anti-psychotic drugs are licensed for the treatment of mania. Their main use is in the treatment of psychosis and they have been shown to reduce or eliminate many of the symptoms of psychosis, such as delusions and hallucinations. In bi-polar disorder, they are used during acute manic episodes to calm the patient, slow racing thoughts and help with sleep. Some of the newer anti-psychotics have mood stabilizing properties. There are a number of different neuroleptics, such as: chlorpromazine (Largactil, Thorazine) haloperidol (Haldol) and trifluoperazine (Stelazine). Newer neuroleptics include risperidone (Risperdal) amisulpride (Solian) and olanzapine (Zyprexa) which are said to have fewer side effects and be easier to take.

Side effects: all of the above drugs are associated with potentially serious side effects and should be used at the lowest effective dose for the shortest time. Side effects include sedation (sleepiness), dry mouth, weight gain, constipation and sensitivity to sunlight. A common class of side effects, the so-called extrapyramidal or parkinsonian side effects, include stiffness and restlessness.

Anti-parkinsonian drugs

These drugs are sometimes given with neuroleptics to relieve side effects. They are not prescribed initially, but only as a treatment for extrapyramidal side-effects if they develop. Anti-parkinsonian drugs include procyclidine (Kemadrin) benzatropine, (Cogentin) and benzhexol/trihexphenidl (Broflex). Side effects of these drugs can include dry mouth, stomach upsets, blurred vision and dizziness.

Minor tranquillisers

These medications, also known as *benzodiazepines* have been used for years to cure anxiety and insomnia. Valium is one of the better known but there are a number of other drugs within the same type. They provide quick relief from anxiety and sleeplessness and, if taken correctly, have fewer side effects. The main problem with these drugs is the risk of dependency. Common benzodiazepines include diazepam (Valium) lorazapam (Ativan) and clonazepam (Rivotril).

Medications and pregnancy

A number of medications for bipolar disorder can be associated with birth defects.

Use effective birth control (contraception) to prevent pregnancy. Discuss birth control options with your doctor, as birth control medications may lose effectiveness when taken along with certain bipolar disorder medications.

If you plan to become pregnant, meet with your doctor to discuss your treatment options.

Discuss breast-feeding with your doctor, as some bipolar medications can pass through breast milk to your infant.

In the next chapter, we will look at professional help and support for those with bi-polar disorder.

Now read the main points from Chapter Three overleaf.

****

Main points from Chapter Three

- The National Institute for Health and Care Excellence (NICE) has guidelines for the treatment of bipolar disorder. They suggest that you should be offered structured psychological treatment while you are relatively stable but may be experiencing mild to moderate symptoms.

- Virtually everyone who has been diagnosed with bipolar disorder will receive medication of one sort or another. Although drugs cannot cure bi-polar disorder they help to manage the symptoms. When starting medication for bi-polar disorder, you should make sure that you know how to take it safely.

- During acute mania or depression you should talk with your doctor at least once a week, or more frequently, to monitor symptoms. As time goes by and you stabilise then you will see your GP less frequently.

****

Chapter 4

Professional Help and Support

In this chapter, we will look at the professional help available for those with bipolar disorder. The range and types of help are many and varied. It is important that you choose the right one for you. In the first instance, bipolar disorder needs to be diagnosed by a psychiatrist, a professional who is medically trained to assess whether someone is suffering from a mental illness. The route to a psychiatrist is through your GP (see below).

Young people and bi-polar

If you are concerned that a young person under 18 may be developing bipolar, it is important to visit your GP and ask for an urgent referral to a specialist. A visit to the Child and Adolescent Mental Health Service (CAMHS) will be necessary, so the young person can be assessed and supported. If the young person is over 18, they will need to ask for help themselves, from their GP.

Early intervention teams can help teenagers and young adults who are at risk of developing psychosis, which can be a feature of bipolar disorder – ask your GP about this service as it is not available in all areas.

If the child or young person is in a very distressed, violent or psychotic state or is at risk of harming themselves or others, you can take them to A&E and ask for an emergency psychiatric assessment. Alternatively you may need to ring the emergency services and ask them to visit the young person at home. They may have to be admitted to hospital under the Mental Health Act, for assessment and treatment.

Young Minds Parents Helpline is there for you if you want to talk about bipolar disorder and how to get your child the best help, Tel 0808 802 5544.
www.youngminds.org.uk/parent/parents-helpline.

General practitioners-the first stop
You're likely to start by seeing your family doctor or a general practitioner. However, in some cases when you call to set up an appointment, you may be referred immediately to a medical doctor who specializes in diagnosing and treating mental health conditions (psychiatrist). Because appointments can be brief, and because there's often a lot of ground to cover, it's a good idea to be well prepared for your appointment. Here's some information to help you get ready for your appointment and know what to expect from your doctor.

What you can do
Write down any symptoms you've had, including any that may seem unrelated to the reason for which you scheduled the

appointment. Write down key personal information, including any major stresses or recent life changes.

Make a list of all medications, vitamins or supplements that you're taking.

Take a family member or friend along, if possible. Sometimes it can be difficult to remember all the information provided to you during an appointment. Someone who accompanies you may remember something that you missed or forgot.

Write down questions to ask your doctor. Your time with your doctor may be limited, so preparing a list of questions ahead of time will help you make the most of your time together. For problems related to bipolar disorder, some basic questions to ask your doctor include:

- Do I have bipolar disorder?
- Are there any other possible causes for my symptoms?
- What kinds of tests will I need?
- What treatments are available? Which do you recommend for me?
- What side effects are possible with that treatment?
- What are the alternatives to the primary approach that you're suggesting?
- I have these other health conditions. How can I best manage these conditions together?
- Should I see a psychiatrist or other mental health provider?

- Is there a generic alternative to the medicine you're prescribing me?
- Are there any brochures or other printed material that I can take home with me? What websites do you recommend visiting?

In addition to the questions that you've prepared to ask your doctor, don't hesitate to ask questions during your appointment at any time that you don't understand something.

What to expect from your doctor
In addition to your questions, your doctor is likely to ask you a number of questions. Being ready to answer them may reserve time to go over any points you want to spend more time on. Your doctor may ask:
- When did you or your loved ones first begin noticing your symptoms of depression, mania or hypomania?
- How frequently do your moods change?
- Do you ever have suicidal thoughts when you're feeling down?
- How severe are your symptoms? Do they interfere with your daily life or relationships?
- Do you have any blood relatives with bi-polar disorder or another mood disorder?
- What other mental or physical health conditions do you have?

- Do you drink alcohol, smoke cigarettes or use street drugs?
- How much do you sleep at night? Does it change over time?
- Do you go through periods when you take risks you wouldn't normally take, such as unsafe sex or unwise, spontaneous financial decisions?
- What, if anything, seems to improve your symptoms?
- What, if anything, appears to worsen your symptoms?

Some alternative treatments may help, but there isn't much research on them. Most of the studies that do exist are on major depression, so it isn't clear how well most of these work for bipolar disorder.

Community mental health teams

If you have been referred to psychiatric services in England or Wales, by your GP, you have a right to get your needs assessed and a care plan developed for you within the Care Programme Approach (CPA). Your care plan should include a thorough assessment of your social and health care needs. You should be allocated a care-coordinator who is in charge of your care and ongoing reviews. You are entitled to say what your needs are and also to have an advocate present. An advocate is someone who can speak for you if necessary.

Often, community care assessments are made by Community Mental Health Teams. Their aim is to help you live independently. They can also help with practical issues, such as sorting out welfare benefits if appropriate and also other services, such as day-centres, or drop in centres. They can also arrange for a Community Psychiatric Nurse (CPN) to visit your home.

Psychotherapy

Psychotherapy is another vital part of bipolar disorder treatment. Several types of therapy may be helpful. These include:

Cognitive behavioral therapy. This is a common form of individual therapy for bipolar disorder. The focus of cognitive behavioral therapy is identifying unhealthy, negative beliefs and behaviors and replacing them with healthy, positive ones. It can help identify what triggers your bipolar episodes. You also learn effective strategies to manage stress and to cope with upsetting situations.

Psychoeducation. Counselling to help you learn about bipolar disorder (psychoeducation) can help you and your loved ones understand bipolar disorder. Knowing what's going on can help you get the best support and treatment, and help you and your loved ones recognize warning signs of mood swings.

Family therapy. Family therapy involves seeing a psychologist or other mental health provider along with your family members. Family therapy can help identify and reduce stress within your family. It can help your family learn how to communicate better, solve problems and resolve conflicts.

Group therapy. Group therapy provides a forum to communicate with and learn from others in a similar situation. It may also help build better relationship skills.

Other therapies. Other therapies that have been studied with some evidence of success include early identification and therapy for worsening symptoms (prodrome detection) and therapy to identify and resolve problems with your daily routine and interpersonal relationships (interpersonal and social rhythm therapy). Ask your doctor if any of these options may be appropriate for you.

Psychodynamic therapists
Psychodynamic theraprists have traditionally viewed psychological and psychiatric problems as originating in a person's childhood and development. Courses of therapy are usually longer than cognitive behavioral therapy, and the therapy may focus less on specific problems and more on personal relationships. Psychodynamic therapists can be dotcors, psychologists or members of other professions. In

addition to being funded by the NHS, it is possible to seek therapy privately.

Care co-ordinators

Over the last few decades, as medications have become more effective, it has become very unusual indeed for people with serious mental illness to spend very long periods in hospital. More and more effeort has gone into helping people to live in the in the community. This approach has had varying degrees of success. In the UK, one key part of this approach, called the care programme approach, calls for certain people to be monitored out in the community by a care co-ordinator who is usually either a nurse or a social worker.

The care coordinator is supposed to meet with the patient regularly, offer advice and support and make sure that he or she is staying well and receiving guidance on taking medication and receiving all other services to which they may be entitled.

If a person is in receipt of benefits, or having financial problems, the care co-ordinator can offer practical support. The care co-ordinator is also supposed to convene regular meetings of all involved with the patient's care, but this will only happen if the illness is very severe.

Hospitalization

In some cases, usually for short periods, people with bipolar disorder benefit from hospitalization. Getting psychiatric treatment at a hospital can help keep you calm and safe and stabilize your mood, whether you're having a manic episode or a deep depression. Partial hospitalization or day treatment programs also are options to consider. These programs provide the support and counselling you need while you get symptoms under control.

Now read the main points from chapter 4 overleaf

***

Main points from chapter 4

- In the first instance, bipolar disorder needs to be diagnosed by a psychiatrist, a professional who is medically trained to assess whether someone is suffering from a mental illness. The route to a psychiatrist is through your GP.

- If you are concerned that a young person under 18 may be developing bipolar, it is important to visit your GP and ask for an urgent referral to a specialist. A visit to the Child and Adolescent Mental Health Service (CAMHS) will be necessary, so the young person can be assessed and supported.

- In some cases when you call to set up an appointment, you may be referred immediately to a medical doctor who specializes in diagnosing and treating mental health conditions (psychiatrist). Because appointments can be brief, and because there's often a lot of ground to cover, it's a good idea to be well prepared for your appointment.

- Often, community care assessments are made by Community Mental Health Teams. Their aim is to help you live independently. They can also help with practical issues, such as sorting out welfare benefits if appropriate and also other services, such as daycentres, or drop in centres. They can also arrange for a community psychiatric nurse (CPN) to visit your home.

- Psychotherapy is another vital part of bipolar disorder treatment. There are a range of therapies.

****

Chapter 5

More about Behavioural Therapies

We discussed the various therapies available to treat bipolar disorder in the last chapter. In this chapter we will expand on cognitive behavioural therapy as it is so important in the treatment of bipolar disorder. As time has gone on, there has been a recognition that mood stabilisers (medications) fail a significant percentage of bi-polar patients.

Therefore, there is room for improving the treatment of bi-polar disorder. Almost all recent developments combine psychotherapy with medication in order to prevent relapses. These approaches are based on assumptions that although medications help the biological aspects of illness, psychotherapy is also needed to help the individual to lead a life that avoids unnecessary stress.

Two types of psychotherapy are being developed for bipolar patients: interpersonal therapy and cognitive behavioural therapy. It is on the latter that we will dwell as interpersonal therapy is still very much in the process of development.

Cognitive Therapy

Cognitive therapy aims to help you to change the way that you think, feel and behave. It is used as a treatment for various mental health and physical problems. Our cognitive processes are our thoughts which include our ideas, mental images, beliefs and attitudes. Cognitive therapy is based on the principle that certain ways of thinking can trigger, or fuel, certain health problems. For example, anxiety, depression, phobias, etc, but there are others, including physical problems. The therapist helps you to understand your current thought patterns. In particular, to identify any harmful, unhelpful, and false ideas or thoughts which you have that can trigger your health problem, or make it worse.

The aim is then to change your ways of thinking to avoid these ideas. Also, to help your thought patterns to be more realistic and helpful.

Behavioural therapy

This aims to change any behaviours that are harmful or not helpful. Various techniques are used. For example, a common unhelpful behaviour is to avoid situations that can make you anxious. In some people with phobias the avoidance can become extreme and affect day-to-day life. In this situation a type of behavioural therapy called exposure therapy may be used. This is where you are gradually exposed more and more to feared situations.

The therapist teaches you how to control anxiety and to cope when you face up to the feared situations.

Cognitive behavioural therapy (CBT)

This is a mixture of cognitive and behavioural therapies. They are often combined because how we behave often reflects how we think about certain things or situations. The emphasis on cognitive or behavioural aspects of therapy can vary, depending on the condition being treated. For example, there is often more emphasis on behavioural therapy when treating obsessive-compulsive disorder (OCD) - where repetitive compulsive actions are a main problem. In contrast, the emphasis may be on cognitive therapy when treating depression.

What conditions can be helped by cognitive behavioural therapy?

CBT has been shown to help people with various conditions - both mental health conditions and physical conditions. As a rule, the more specific the problem, the more likely CBT may help. This is because it is a practical therapy which focuses on particular problems and aims to overcome them. CBT is sometimes used alone, and sometimes used in addition to medication, depending on the type and severity of the condition being treated.

What is likely to happen during a course of cognitive behavioural therapy?

The first session of therapy will usually include time for the therapist and you to develop a shared understanding of the problem. This is usually to identify how your thoughts, ideas, feelings, attitudes, and behaviours affect your day-to-day life. You should then agree a treatment plan and goals to achieve, and the number of sessions likely to be needed. Each session lasts about 50-60 minutes. Typically, a session of therapy is done once a week. Most courses of CBT last for several weeks. It is common to have 10-15 sessions, but a course of CBT can be longer or shorter, depending on the nature and severity of the condition. In some situations, CBT sessions can be done by telephone.

You have to take an active part and are given homework between sessions. For example, if you have social phobia, early in the course of therapy you may be asked to keep a diary of your thoughts which occur when you become anxious before a social event. Later on you may be given homework to try out ways of coping which you have learned during therapy.

How well does cognitive behavioural therapy work?
CBT has been shown in clinical trials to help ease symptoms of various health problems. For example, research studies have shown that a course of CBT is just as likely to be effective as medication in treating depression and certain anxiety disorders. There may be long-term benefits of CBT, as the techniques to combat these problems can be used for the rest of your life to help to keep symptoms away. So, for example, depression or anxiety are less likely to recur in the future.

CBT is one type of psychotherapy (talking treatment). Unlike other types of psychotherapy, it does not involve talking freely, or dwell on events in your past to gain insight into your emotional state of mind. It is not a "lie on the couch and tell all" type of therapy.

CBT tends to deal with the here and now - how your current thoughts and behaviours are affecting you now. It recognises that events in your past have shaped the way that you currently think and behave. In particular, thought patterns and behaviours learned in childhood, However, CBT does not dwell on the past, but aims to find solutions to how to change your current thoughts and behaviours so that you can function better now and in the future.

CBT is also different to counselling, which is meant to be non-directive, empathetic and supportive. Although the CBT therapist will offer support and empathy, the therapy has a structure, is problem-focused and practical.

What are the limitations of cognitive behavioural therapy?

CBT does not suit everyone and it is not helpful for all conditions. You need to be committed and persistent in tackling and improving your health problem with the help of the therapist. It can be hard work. The homework may be difficult and challenging. You may be taken 'out of your comfort zone' when tackling situations which cause anxiety or distress. However, many people have greatly benefited from a course of CBT.

How can I get cognitive behavioural therapy?

Your doctor may refer you to a therapist who has been trained in CBT. This may be a psychologist, psychiatrist, psychiatric nurse, or other healthcare professional. There is a limited number of CBT therapists available on the NHS. You may wish to go privately if it is not available in your area on the NHS. However, government policy is to make CBT more widely available on the NHS.

Do-it-yourself cognitive behavioural therapy

Although CBT with the help of a trained therapist is best, some people prefer to tackle their problems themselves. There are a range of books and leaflets on self-help for the problems which CBT is useful for (anxiety, phobias, depression, etc). More recently, interactive CDs and websites are being developed and evaluated for self-directed CBT for a variety of conditions.

In the next chapter, we will be taking a look of the effects of stigma and shame on bipolar sufferers and how to deal with this.

Now read the main points from Chapter 5 overleaf

****

Main points from chapter 5

- As time has gone on, there has been a recognition that mood stabilisers (medications) fail a significant percentage of bipolar patients. Therefore, there is room for improving the treatment of bipolar disorder.

- Almost all recent developments combine psychotherapy with medication in order to prevent relapses. These approaches are based on assumptions that although medications help the biological aspects of illness, psychotherapy is also needed to help the individual to lead a life that avoids unnecessary stress.

- Cognitive Behavioural Therapy (CBT) aims to help you to change the way that you think, feel and behave. It is used as a treatment for various mental health and physical problems.

- Your doctor may refer you to a therapist who has been trained in CBT. This may be a psychologist, psychiatrist, psychiatric nurse, or other healthcare professional. There is a limited number of CBT therapists available on the NHS. You may wish to go privately if it is not available in your area on the NHS.

****

Chapter 6

Dealing With Stigma and Shame

Bipolar- Stigmatisation and Feelings of Shame
Illnesses generally cause distress and discomfort, including physical pain and mental discomfort. However, some illnesses, such as bipolar disorder can cause additional problems by affecting the way we feel about ourselves around other people. Sufferers may feel ashamed or embarrassed to admit their diagnoses because of the reactions of others.

Everyone should have the right to decide when and with whom to disclose health problems. In some cases, privacy can be both appropriate and desirable. There is a difference, however, between illnesses we choose to keep private simply out of personal preference and those that we feel we must keep private in order to preserve our social standing, our jobs or our legal rights. When we feel that we have to keep our illness a secret, as do many with psychological disorders, we are feeling the effects of stigma.

Stigma
Stigma is a term used to describe two things, a feeling of prejudice or dislike towards some group on the part of the

general population, and the corresponding feeling of shame caused in that group by that prejudice. The stigmatisation of the mentally ill is rife and has been much studied. This stigmatisation is caused by ignorance and fear of outsiders, those who do not suffer from bipolar disorder.

Effects of stigma

Stigma seems to affect sufferers in two ways: through their reaction to others and through their feelings about themselves. Some sufferers worry about the reaction of others, fearing that they might not be accepted, or that other people will think of them as 'mad'. Alternatively, some people are more affected by internal feelings of shame and worthlessness, the feeling that they are deeply flawed.

Inner feelings of stigmatisation can produce a sense of low self-worth: you may feel damaged or inferior in some way. Such a feeling can be combated in various ways and careful thought about one's own personal state is necessary.

Plenty of illnesses, including HIV and hepatitis, can be stigmatising. When it comes to mental disorders, however, stigma and shame can operate in a couple of unique ways.

Those with common psychological disorders, especially depression and anxiety, frequently feel bad about themselves to begin with. That's one of the primary identifying symptoms of these illnesses. Therefore, stigma about mental illness feeds into their psychological symptoms, which can in turn worsen feelings of stigma and shame.

Depression, anxiety and bipolar disorder can cause people to behave in ways that they usually wouldn't. They might miss or break important appointments. They can be more irritable and impatient with loved ones and treat them badly. They might drink more, take drugs, spend compulsively, or engage in other obsessive behaviours. Often, they try to keep their worst behaviour a secret from those around them. All of this exacerbates underlying feelings of shame and guilt and can cause others to judge them harshly.

When all of this is taken together, it is completely understandable if we want to tell no one about our illness. Unfortunately, trying to cope with mental illness without the help and support of others can hinder our recovery and keep us from getting care we might need.

The first step away from the negative feedback loop of stigma and shame comes in the form of information, information about how common psychological problems are, how effective treatment can be, and how likely it is that those with mental disorders will lead rich and fulfilling lives.

Another important step is seeking qualified help. Effective treatment-psychological, medical and social-makes a huge difference in terms of our symptoms and how we feel about ourselves. Receiving a formal diagnosis of a mental disorder might bring up feelings of stigma and shame. Some people fear that this forever marks them as different from everyone else, or that they can never lead a normal and happy life. This doesn't have to be the case.

A diagnosis is a label that professionals use to help determine the proper course of treatment. The diagnosis, however, doesn't define you. It defines the problem and how you and your doctor can combat it.

Telling people you trust about your problem will also help fight stigma and shame. This can start with your primary health care provider or your mental health care provider. Ultimately, sharing what you've been through with close friends and family, or with other people who have struggled with the same illness, can be both a freeing and healing experience. Disclosure must be approached cautiously, but it can be an effective tool not only to break out of isolation, but also to restore feelings of self-confidence.

Freedom from stigma can also come from examining your life and values then figuring out how to overcome your limitations and give back to the world in a way that is meaningful to you. For some, this might mean spending more time with children or grandchildren or helping friends and neighbours. For others, it might mean engaging in volunteer or church work. Still others find satisfaction and fulfilment in telling their story more publicly or in helping others who are struggling with mental illness. Ultimately, the more that people like us talk openly about our illness, the more that stigma will fade away-not just from our own lives, but also from society at large.

Finally, of course bi-polar disorder can be a disabling and distressing illness. In this it is similar to many other disabilities. few people would choose to be blind or without a limb but this does not mean that a disabled person is of less worth than others. A humane society, which hopefully we are in, is one with opportunity for all.

In the final analysis, the best way of combating the sense of stigma is to first obtain all the help that you can, and then to work to make your life as fulfilled as possible. There is a lot people with bipolar can do to diminish the bad effects of the illness and lead fulfilling lives.

In the next chapter, we will look at bipolar disorder and the nature and effect of vicious cycles.

Now read the main points from Chapter 6 overleaf

****

Main *points from Chapter 6*

- Illnesses generally cause distress and discomfort, including physical pain and mental discomfort. However, some illnesses, such as bipolar disorder can cause additional problems by affecting the way we feel about ourselves around other people. Stigmatisation and shame may arise as a result of these negative feelings.

- Inner feelings of stigmatisation can produce a sense of low self-worth: you may feel damaged or inferior in some way. Such a feeling can be combated in various ways and careful thought about one's own personal state is necessary.

- The first step away from the negative feedback loop of stigma and shame comes in the form of information, information about how common psychological problems are, how effective treatment can be, and how likely it is that those with mental disorders will lead rich and fulfilling lives.

- In the final analysis, the best way of combating the sense of stigma is to first obtain all the help that you can, and then to work to make your life as fulfilled as possible.

****

Chapter 7

Bipolar Disorder and Vicious Cycles

Bipolar Disorder and Vicious Cycles

Vicious cycles are often found to play an important role in a variety of everyday psychological problems, but especially in bipolar disorder. This is when one thing leads to another and then back again. For example, in alcoholics, one drink may lead to another and another, and afterward they feel ashamed or depressed, only to use that as an excuse to start drinking again. Then it's like a vicious cycle, repeating itself.

This can happen to people with bipolar disorder as well. For example, procrastination is a very common problem for people with the disorder. Procrastination can also set up a vicious cycle – the more you delay dealing with your problems and tasks, the more difficult they begin to seem, so you put off doing them further, which is more procrastination.

This happens during bipolar episodes, someone in a manic episode can feel powerful, attractive, successful, etc. Because they "feel" energetic, they decline the need for sleep. Then sleep deprivation makes the manic episode worse, and they are in a vicious cycle. On the other hand, someone in a depressive episode can feel worthless, helpless, hopeless, likely to fail, etc.

This leads to inactivity, more sleep, and isolation, which are all triggers for episodes, so the vicious cycle continues.

The first step to breaking out of a vicious cycle is to recognize that you are in one.

Vicious cycles and stress

As we have seen in the earlier chapters, stress is the enemy of the person with bipolar disorder. Life is stressful enough for everyone, particularly in this modern age where housing and employment is becoming more difficult to access and life in general is harder than it was. Although a certain amount of stress can be positive, it is where the stress becomes excessive that leads to vicious cycles. You might be faced with multiple demands, feel anxious, nervous and tense and you might procrastinate and not meet these demands, which leads you into a vicious cycle as the situation can only get worse.

The first thing that you have to do is to make sure that you are organised and that everything is down in black and white and that you can follow your script-i.e. you have a list of things that you need to do and do them, to avoid problems piling up.

Relaxation

Stress can cause all sorts of problems, not least physical. problems can include excessive sweating, restlessness, stomach problems and rapid heartbeat. Stress can also lead to lack of sleep due to worry the best way to combat these particular side effects is by adopting certain relaxation techniques. A variety of tried and tested techniques can be used.

Breathing Exercise

This relaxation technique can be very a potent weapon against anxiety or panic attacks. it can also be used during a manic phase of Bipolar disorder. Doing this exercise before laying down to go to sleep may help with insomnia in some people.

When experiencing a panic attack, it is best, if possible, to close your mouth and breathe through your nose to avoid hyperventilation.

It is also advisable any time you practice breathing exercises to either sit or lie down to prevent passing out or falling due to dizziness.

Many people find it useful to do these exercises before they begin visualization, or meditation to help them relax. Also, many people find positive self-talk useful in conjunction with these exercises. Such as calmly saying short phrases like " Let it go" or "It's all ok " silently to yourself while exhaling.

The idea is to get yourself to relax as much as possible. Trying to relax or judge your performance may be counter-productive, so clear your mind of everything except your positive self talk or counting between breaths.

Note the amount of tension you are feeling, and let it go as much as possible while exhaling slowly through your nose or mouth. (Again, if you are having a panic attack, it is best to keep your mouth closed.) Then breathe slowly and deeply into your abdomen. (You will know you are doing this correctly if you place your hand on your abdomen and feel it rising as you breathe in.) Hold the breath for a count of 2-5 seconds (whatever you are more comfortable with. The longer you hold the more you will relax when you exhale, but to prevent passing out you should not hold it any longer than 5 seconds)

Exhale again, slowly for anywhere between 5 and 10 seconds. Repeat breathing this way until your anxiety subsides, or you feel properly relaxed.

Progressive Muscle Relaxation

If you have anxiety disorder it is advisable to do this exercise every day. When you start out , it is best to do this for around 20 minutes. As you gain skill in relaxation technique the amount of time you need will diminish. Find a quiet place to practice in. If you feel the need to play music, choose relaxing instrumental music. If you play music that has lyrics, it may distract you, or work to govern your mood.   Try to do this at the same time every day. If you suffer from insomnia, you may find it helpful to do this before bed.

Make sure you are neither hungry nor overfull. Also make sure you are in a comfortable position, wearing comfortable clothing, and you take off your shoes, jewellery, glasses, contacts, etc. Make a decision to not worry about anything during this time. Make peace of mind for this amount of time a priority every day. As with the breathing exercise, it is not necessary to judge your performance or try to relax. This is your time every day to just "let go". Once you are comfortable and relaxed, (you may want to do the breathing exercise first) start by curling and tensing your toes. Tense them hard enough to feel it, but not hard enough that you feel strained. Hold the tension for about ten seconds, concentrating on how it feels and then let it go. Stop for a moment to notice the difference between how they felt when they were tensed and how they feel relaxed.

Next, curl and tense your feet, concentrate on how they feel, hold the tension for about 10 seconds and release. Notice the difference. Next tense your calves, continue this process of tensing and releasing the muscles all the way up your body, thighs, buttocks, abdomen, back,(by gently arching it) fists, lower arms, upper arms, shoulders, neck,(by gently lifting your head, holding it up and then gently laying it back down)and face (scrunch it up ... nobody is looking). Repeat this process beginning with your face and progressing back down to your toes. Now would be a good time to also repeat the breathing exercise.

Visualization
After completing the breathing and progressive muscle relaxation exercises, you may want to do some visualization. This is a bit like meditation.

Design a peaceful scene for yourself. It may be helpful to write it out on a piece of paper and study it before you begin. Your scene can be anywhere you choose. At home in front of a cosy fire, or at the ocean. It's up to you. The only thing you need to worry about, is that there is enough detail involved in your scene to absorb your full attention.

Here is an example:
I am lying on a soft grassy spot along the bank of a rushing river in the woods. It is a warm summer evening at dusk. There is a purple ribbon of colour just above a mountain as the sun finishes setting behind it. I can hear the water rushing beside me and feel a slight mist of water spraying over me in contrast to the warm breeze that is blowing the fragrance of water, pine and wildflowers over me as well. I can hear birds chirping in the tall pine trees, and the wood crackling in the campfire that is burning not too far away. As I watch the smoke rising from the campfire into the navy-blue sky, I begin to see stars appearing overhead.

You may wish to record your peaceful scene onto a tape so that you can visualize it without effort. After you become comfortable with returning to your scene, you can practice going there to do your progressive muscle relaxation or breathing exercises.

Again, doing this every day will be helpful with reducing stress and helping you relax. Doing these relaxation exercises before bedtime, may help reduce the symptoms of insomnia.

The vicious cycle of anger and controlling anger

Expressing anger is a normal human emotion that everyone experiences to varying degrees. Bipolar Disorder sufferers, however, are especially prone to experiencing extreme mood swings, changeable behaviour patterns and irritable symptoms because this combination is a prominent aspect of the disorder. Accepting the emotional challenges that compromise behaviour, when living with bipolar disorder, may help achieve better understanding of the anger expressed.

Understanding Your Anger Pattern

If you live with bipolar disorder, then you will understand only too well that the mild or severe shift in mood impacts on everyday life and can create aggressive and excessive behaviour and also depressive symptoms. This negative pattern affects individuals in many ways and severe agitation and anger may also develop during manic periods.

It is very important indeed to clearly identify your anger pattern. By doing so you will be more able to avoid negative triggers and to create positive changes where appropriate. You will also be able to understand how stress and life events affect you, and how fear and resentment also play a part in maintaining a negative outlook. Once you are able to understand your anger pattern you will be able to learn ways of alternative responses. One of the most important responses is to stop and reflect, if possible, take a deep breath and draw back. Quite often, during episodes of mania, sudden anger will lead to actions that cause regret, can even lead to grave problems after the event.

Suppressing Anger

Viewing things and situations from a negative perspective is both destructive and restrictive. Bipolar disorder predisposes sufferers to manic behaviour symptoms that can create continually negative patterns of mood swing that impact on anger, stress and frustration. If these emotions are suppressed in a negative manner, through bottling up and turning feelings inwards, the outcome and consequences become more escalated and unmanageable. If, however, anger is channelled in a constructive and positive way the extreme emotions can become easier to manage.

Learning to express feelings in a calm manner is healthy and important in making improvements in the effective, positive suppression of anger. Using calming strategies with the aid of relaxation and breathing techniques as described above, will help to reduce inner turmoil and maintain neutral behaviour. Exercising regularly and using visualisation techniques, during relaxation periods, also works well in creating a positive change in behaviour.

To summarise, things you and/or your partner can do to minimise the impact of vicious cycles are:
1. Avoid stress – this is the biggest trigger to a vicious cycle.

2. Stay active.
3. Be productive – but not excessively.
4. Communicate with each other.
5. Help each other recognize the other one's vicious cycles.
6. Consciously face the vicious cycle.
7. Replace negative thoughts with positive thoughts.
8. Think all the way through things before you do them.

The more you and/or your spouse can make fighting vicious cycles a conscious thing, the better off you will be, instead of just reacting, or acting impulsively, which makes a vicious cycle worse.

In the next chapter, we will deal with one other important element in dealing with vicious cycles that is well worth mentioning, and that is an understanding of **assertiveness** and how this impacts on you as an individual.

Now read the main points from Chapter 7 overleaf.

****

Main points from chapter 7

- Vicious cycles are often found to play an important role in a variety of everyday psychological problems, but especially in bipolar disorder. This is when one thing leads to another and then back again. For example, in alcoholics, one drink may lead to another and another, and afterward they feel ashamed or depressed, only to use that as an excuse to start drinking again. Then it's like a vicious cycle, repeating itself.

- Procrastination is a very common problem for people with the disorder. Procrastination can also set up a vicious cycle – the more you delay dealing with your problems and tasks, the more difficult they begin to seem, so you put off doing them further, which is more procrastination.

- Stress can cause all sorts of problems, not least physical. problems can include excessive sweating, restlessness, stomach problems and rapid heartbeat. Stress can also lead to lack of sleep due to worry the best way to combat these particular side effects is by adopting certain relaxation techniques. A variety of tried and tested techniques can be used such as breathing exercises and progressive muscle relaxation.

- Anger is one emotion that gives rise to a vicious cycle and must be controlled.

****

Chapter 8

Assertiveness-The Importance of Being Assertive in the Control of Vicious Cycles

---

Understanding the concept of assertiveness and the need for bipolar sufferers in particular to be assertive but not aggressive is essential to controlling situations and avoiding vicious cycles.

Assertiveness is not a personality trait which persists consistently across all situations. Different individuals exhibit varying degrees of assertive behaviour depending on whether they are in a work, social, academic, recreational or relationship context.

The most important point to remember is that there is a big difference between being assertive and standing up for yourself and being aggressive.

Non-Assertiveness

A non-assertive person is one who is often taken advantage of, feels helpless, takes on everyone's problems, says yes to inappropriate demands and thoughtless requests, and allows others to choose for him or her. However, the non-assertive person can get angry if he or she feels ignored or in any way a victim of injustice.

The non-assertive person is emotionally dishonest, indirect, self-denying, and inhibited. He/she feels hurt, anxious, and possibly angry about his/her actions.

Non-Assertive Body Language:
- Lack of eye contact; looking down or away.
- Swaying and shifting of weight from one foot to the other.
- Whining and hesitancy when speaking.

Assertiveness

An assertive person is one who acts in his/her own best interests, stands up for self, expresses feelings honestly, is in charge of self in interpersonal relations, and chooses for self.

An assertive person is emotionally honest, direct, self-enhancing, and expressive. He/she feels confident, self-respecting at the time of his/her actions as well as later. There is a big difference between being assertive and being aggressive.

Assertive Body Language:
- Stand straight, steady, and directly face the people to whom you are speaking while maintaining eye contact.
- Speak in a clear, steady voice - loud enough for the people to whom you are speaking to hear you.
- Speak fluently, without hesitation, and with assurance and confidence.

Aggressiveness

An aggressive person is one who wins by using power, hurts others, is intimidating, controls the environment to suit his/her needs, and chooses for others.

He/she is inappropriately expressive, emotionally honest, direct, and self-enhancing at the expense of another. An aggressive person feels righteous, superior, deprecatory at the time of action and possibly guilty later.

Aggressive Body Language:
- Leaning forward with glaring eyes.
- Pointing a finger at the person to whom you are speaking.
- Shouting.
- Clenching the fists.
- Putting hands on hips and wagging the head.
-

How To Improve the Communication Process
- Active listening: reflecting back (paraphrasing) to the other person
- Identifying your position: stating your thoughts and feelings about the situation.

Assertive Ways of Saying "No":
Basic principles to follow in answers:
- brevity, clarity, firmness, and honesty.

- Begin your answer with the word "NO" so it is not ambiguous.
- Make your answer short and to the point.
- Don't give a long explanation.
- Be honest, direct and firm.
- Don't say, "I'm sorry, but..."

The above is just an outline of assertiveness techniques. It is very wise to give a lot of thought to your approach to anger management and also assertiveness techniques. There are lots of organisations offering advice in this area and several are listed in the useful addresses and websites section at the end of this book.

In the next chapter, we will explore the risks of sleep loss and its effects on bipolar disorder.

Now read the main points from Chapter 8 overleaf

****

Main points from Chapter 8

- Understanding the concept of assertiveness and the need for bi-polar sufferers in particular to be assertive but not aggressive is essential to controlling situations and avoiding vicious cycles.

- The most important point to remember is that there is a big difference between being assertive and standing up for yourself and being aggressive.

- A non-assertive person is one who is often taken advantage of, feels helpless, takes on everyone's problems, says yes to inappropriate demands and thoughtless requests, and allows others to choose for him or her.

- An assertive person is one who acts in his/her own best interests, stands up for self, expresses feelings honestly, is in charge of self in interpersonal relations, and chooses for self.

- An aggressive person is one who wins by using power, hurts others, is intimidating, controls the environment to suit his/her needs, and chooses for others.

- Being assertive will help enormously in the process of combating vicious cycles and also achieving self-confidence.

****

Chapter 9

The Risks of Sleep Loss

We have established at the beginning of this book how important sleep is to the maintenance of the health of bipolar sufferers. Many people have problems with sleep, some more than others. However, for those with bipolar disorder sleep is of the utmost importance. This can be a vicious circle as the very fact that a person suffers from bipolar often means that sleep patterns will be disturbed.

How bipolar disorder affects sleep
Bipolar disorder may affect sleep in many ways. For example, it can lead to:
- Insomnia: this is the inability to fall asleep or remain asleep long enough to feel rested.
- Delayed sleep phase syndrome, a circadian-rhythm sleep disorder resulting in insomnia and daytime sleepiness.
- REM (rapid eye movement) sleep abnormalities, which may make dreams very vivid or bizarre.
- Irregular sleep-wake schedules, which sometimes results from a lifestyle that involves medication-seeking behaviour at night.

During the lows of bipolar disorder, you may have overwhelming feelings of hopelessness, sadness and worthlessness. These can interfere with your sleep. During the highs of bipolar disorder (periods of mania), you may be so aroused that you can go for days without sleep. For three in four people with bipolar disorder, sleep problems are the most common signal that a period of mania is about to occur. When sleep is in short supply, someone with bipolar disorder may not miss it the way other people would. However, even though you seem to get by on so little sleep, lack of sleep can take quite a toll. For example, you may:
- Be extremely moody
- Feel sick, tired, depressed or worried
- Have trouble concentrating or making decisions
- Be at higher risk of an accidental death
- Get better sleep with bipolar disorder.

Disrupted sleep can really aggravate a mood disorder. A first step might involve figuring out all the factors that may be affecting sleep and discussing them with the doctor.

Keeping a sleep diary may help. Include information about:
- How long it takes to go to sleep
- How many times you wake up during the night
- How long you sleep all night

- When you take medication or use caffeine, alcohol or nicotine
- When you exercise and for how long.

Certain bipolar medications may also affect sleep as a side effect. For example, they may disrupt the sleep-wake cycle. One way to address this is to move bedtime and waking time later and later each day until you reach your desired goal. Another way to handle this situation is with bright light therapy.

Of course, your doctor may recommend a change in medication if needed. Be sure to discuss any other medicines or medical conditions that may be affecting your sleep, such as arthritis, migraines or a back injury.

Restoring a regular schedule of daily activities and sleep - perhaps with the help of cognitive behavioural therapy - can go a long way towards helping restore more even moods.

Ways to get better sleep

A lot of people have trouble sleeping from time to time. However, you can make it easier to get a good night's sleep every night with these simple steps:
- *Cut caffeine.* Caffeine can keep you awake. It can stay in your body longer than you might think - the effects of caffeine can take as long as eight hours to wear off. So if you drink a cup of coffee in the afternoon and are still tossing at night, caffeine might be the reason. Cutting out

caffeine at least four to six hours before bedtime can help you fall asleep more easily.
- *Avoid alcohol* as a sleep aid. Alcohol may initially help you fall asleep, but it also causes disturbances in sleep resulting in less restful sleep. An alcoholic drink before bedtime may make it more likely that you will wake up during the night.
- *Relax before bedtime.* Stress not only makes you miserable, it wreaks havoc on your sleep. Develop some kind of pre-sleep ritual to break the connection between all the day's stress and bedtime. These rituals can be as short as 10 minutes or as long as an hour. Some people find relief in making a list of all the stressful things that have happened during the day, along with a plan to deal with them. This can act as "closure" to the day. Combining this with a period of relaxation perhaps by reading something light, meditating, aromatherapy, light stretching or taking a hot bath can also help you get better sleep. Also, don't look at the clock!
- *Exercise at the right time for you.* Regular exercise can help you get a good night's sleep. The timing and intensity of exercise seems to play a key role in its effects on sleep. If you are the type of person who gets energised or becomes more alert after exercise, it may be best not to exercise in the evening. Regular exercise in

the morning even can help relieve insomnia, according to a study.

- *Keep your bedroom quiet*, dark and comfortable. For many people, even the slightest noise or light can disturb sleep like the purring of a cat or the light from your laptop or TV. Consider using earplugs, window blinds or curtains and an electric blanket - everything possible to create an ideal sleep environment. Don't use the overhead light if you need to get up at night; use a small night-light instead. Ideal room temperatures for sleeping are between 15C and 22C (59F and 71F). Temperatures above 24C (75F) or below about 12C (53F) can disrupt sleep.
- *Eat right, sleep tight.* Try not to go to bed hungry but avoid heavy meals before bedtime. An over-full stomach can keep you up, but some people believe certain foods can help. Milk contains tryptophan, which limited research suggests may, but is not proven to be, a sleep-promoting chemical or natural sedative. Foods like poultry, bananas, oats and honey contain tryptophan. Carbohydrate-rich foods like bread and crackers may complement dairy foods like milk, by increasing the level of tryptophan in the blood. Meanwhile, try not to drink fluids after 8pm. This can keep you from having to get up to use the toilet.

- *Restrict nicotine.* Having a smoke before bed - although it feels relaxing actually puts a stimulant into your bloodstream. The effects of nicotine are similar to those of caffeine. Nicotine can keep you up and awaken you at night. It should be avoided particularly near bedtime and if you wake up in the middle of the night.
- *Avoid napping.* Napping may make matters worse if you usually have problems falling asleep.
- *Keep pets off the bed.* If a pet sleeps with you then this, too, may cause you to awaken during the night, either from allergies or pet movements. Fido and Fluffy might be better off on the floor than on your sheets.
- *Avoid watching TV*, eating and discussing emotional issues in bed. The bed should be used for sleep (and sex) only. If not, you can end up associating the bed with distracting activities that could make it difficult for you to fall asleep.

In the next chapter we will look at bipolar and issues within the family.

Now read the main points from Chapter 9 overleaf

****

Main points from Chapter 9

- Bipolar disorder may affect sleep in many ways. For example it can lead to insomnia, delayed sleep phase syndrome, REM (rapid eye movement) and irregular sleep-wake schedules.

- Disrupted sleep can really aggravate a mood disorder. A first step might involve figuring out all the factors that may be affecting sleep and discussing them with the doctor. Keeping a sleep diary may help.

- A lot of people have trouble sleeping from time to time. However, you can make it easier to get a good night's sleep every night with simple steps as described in chapter 9.

****

Chapter 10

Bipolar Disorder-Family Issues

If you have been diagnosed with bipolar disorder, your family will be involved right from the outset. Having bipolar disorder will not prevent you from leaving home, and it is a fact that most sufferers manage to leave home and live independent lives. Some people have managed to maintain stable relationships. However, whatever the circumstance, it is almost certain that family will stay involved. Sometimes, this involvement arises out of feelings of guilt because family feel that they may have passed the problem on genetically.

Although parental support can be very welcome in the first instance, particularly helping a person access appropriate care at the beginning of the illness, it can be difficult determining levels of involvement as time moves on. Over-involvement can cause resentment in the sufferer, particularly if the sufferer perceives this involvement as interference in their life. It can be a difficult balance to strike.

With younger adults, parents will no doubt be concerned with a person's social competence in managing money and dealing with friends and also issues such as employment and dealing with others generally. Parents can also be concerned about sexuality, as a young person with bipolar may be vulnerable which can lead to unprotected sex, and the attendant problems with this, such as AIDS and other diseases.

Over-vigilance can be counter productive and it is probably best for parents and the person suffering from bipolar to discuss openly the problems and the best ways to tackle them. If this cannot, for some reason, be achieved then there are professional counsellors who will assist with the process. See the useful addresses at the back of the book.

Involvement of spouses and partners

Spouses and partners of bipolar sufferers are directly involved on a day-to-day basis. However, they also have their own feelings to cope with at the same time. Some spouses or partners may have formed a relationship with a bipolar sufferer in the full knowledge that they have that condition and accepted this as a 'part of the package'. However, from experience, in many cases it has to be said that bipolar disorder becomes apparent after people get together and this causes complications.

Grief and anger can arise, for both partners, as the problem unfolds and it becomes obvious that the future that you had envisaged together will not go according to plan. There can also be feelings of anger and resentment if one person feels that they weren't informed by the other that a condition existed. It is very important, even crucial, for both partners to respect the views of each other and to try to work through problems and arrive at a form of communication between each other. This will help provide a resolution to the problems that have arisen or are unfolding.

There are many support groups out there which will prove crucial in the maintenance of relationships between couples. These groups often consist of people who have been though the experience and can pass on first hand knowledge.

Family members, whether spouse, partner or parent can have a vital role in helping sufferers notice early signs of episodes so that they can use psychological skills to avert further problems or seek help from their mental health team. However, a balance needs to be drawn between this positive role and the risk of friction between family members if they are seen to be over-sensitive to even small changes in the behaviour of the person with bi-polar disorder. This balance involves a recognition that all people experience fluctuating mood states, including anger, happiness, frustration boredom and excitement. Thus, evidence of irritability in someone with bi-polar disorder is not necessarily a sign of anything other than their being irritated by an event in a normal way.

Family breakdown after illness and rebuilding relationships
In bipolar disorder there are two types of problem that can affect sufferers and their families. Having to cope with the problems of both depression and mania can be harder to

understand for carers and spouses than dealing with depression in isolation. These episodes can cause significant problems for the family. Some symptoms of both depression and mania can be perceived as malicious and intentional. This is where real problems can start and can cause rifts and break up of relationships.

Sufferers are always advised to attempt to rebuild relationships that have suffered as a result of these episodes, when they are well. Also, clinical professionals may be crucial here in helping families understand and to be educated about the nature of the episodes and realise that they are not malicious but are a result of the condition.

It is advised that, when the sufferer is well, they should put in as much time as possible in rebuilding trust and repairing damaged relationships and also mending ill-feelings.

At times, a family can be particularly resentful if they perceive an episode as having been triggered by a sufferer's stopping his or her mood stabilisers. In this case, families see their sick relative as being irresponsible. Family education is important here which involves professionals. They will make it clear that sometimes it is hard to judge whether sufferers stopped taking medication and then relapsed or whether they were in an early state of relapse when they stopped taking medication.

Families will almost certainly feel resentful if they see their relative or spouse abusing their selves with alcohol or drugs which fly's in the face of good advice. It is up to family to put their foot down if this happens and point out that this type of counter-productive behaviour is jeopardising their relationship with each other.

Now read the main points from chapter 10 overleaf.

****

Main points from Chapter 10

- If you have been diagnosed with bipolar disorder, your family will be involved right from the outset

- Although parental support can be very welcome in the first instance, particularly helping a person access appropriate care at the beginning of the illness, it can be difficult determining levels of involvement as time moves on.

- Spouses and partners of bipolar sufferers are directly involved on a day-to-day basis. However, they also have their own feelings to cope with at the same time

- Grief and anger can arise, for both partners, as the problem unfolds and it becomes obvious that the future that you had envisaged together will not go according to plan.

- It is very important, even crucial, for both partners to respect the views of each other and to try to work through problems and arrive at a form of communication between each other. This will help provide a resolution to the problems that have arisen or are unfolding.

- There are many support groups out there that will prove crucial in the maintenance of relationships between couples and other family members.

Chapter 11

Bi-Polar Disorder and Diet

Is there a specific diet for people with Bipolar Disorder?

The first thing to emphasise is that there is no specific bipolar diet. Nevertheless, it is very important indeed to make wise dietary choices that will help you maintain a healthy weight and stay well. This applies to all people, whether bipolar sufferers or not.

These choices include:
- Avoiding the "Western" style diet that is rich in red meats, saturated fats and trans-fat and simple carbohydrates. This eating style is linked to a higher risk for obesity, type 2 diabetes, and heart disease. Eating less saturated fats and simple carbohydrates can help overall health but does not directly affect the symptoms of bipolar disorder.
- Eating a balance of protective, nutrient-dense foods. These foods include fresh fruits, vegetables, legumes, whole grains, lean meats, cold-water fish, eggs, low-fat dairy, soy products, and nuts and seeds.

- These foods provide the levels of nutrients necessary to maintain good health and prevent disease.
- Watching caloric intake and exercising regularly to maintain a healthy weight. Some findings show that those with bipolar disorder may have a greater risk of being overweight or obese. Talk to your doctor about ways to avoid weight gain when taking bipolar medications.

Does Fish Oil Improve Mood With Bipolar Disorder?

It is generally acknowledged that eating fatty fish at least two times a week is good for most people. Good choices include:
- Albacore tuna
- Herring
- Mackerel
- Salmon
- Trout

If you do not like fish, it is recommended that you take 0.5 to 1.8 grams of fish oil per day as supplements. That way you will get enough eicosapentaenoic acid (EPA) and docosahexaenoic acid (DHA).

Fish oil can help keep your heart healthy. But some experts also believe that fish oil is an important bipolar supplement and that it plays a key role in brain function and behaviour. These experts report that omega-3 fatty acids may be helpful for those with bipolar disorder, particularly if they have an higher risk of cardiovascular disease or high triglycerides.

Some research suggests that getting more omega-3 fatty acids found in fish oil is linked to greater volume in areas of the brain. In particular, these areas are related to mood and behaviour. Results from one study of 75 patients describe the benefits of omega-3 fatty acids compared to a placebo. The benefits included decreasing depression in bipolar disorder.

If you're a vegetarian or vegan looking for possible benefits of fish oil, go with nuts. Walnuts, flaxseed, and canola oil contain alpha-linolenic acid (ALA), which is converted to omega-3 fatty acid in the body.

Which Foods to Avoid for bi-polar sufferers

Some general dietary recommendations for treating bipolar disorder include:
- Getting only moderate amounts of caffeine and not stopping caffeine use abruptly
- Avoiding high-fat meals to lower the risk for obesity
- Watching your salt if you have high blood pressure but not skimping on salt if you are being prescribed lithium since low salt intake can cause higher levels of lithium in the blood
- Following your doctor's instructions to stay away from foods that may affect your specific bipolar medication, if any.

In addition, you need to be wary of natural dietary supplements that can cause a drug-herb interaction.

Avoiding too much Caffeine may be helpful for getting good sleep, which is especially important for people with bipolar disorder. When someone with bipolar disorder is feeling depressed, extra caffeine can help that person boost the low mood. The problem is caffeine can disrupt sleep. Caffeine can also lower the sedative effects of medications, such as benzodiazepines, that are used to treat anxiety and mania associated with bipolar disorder.

In addition to lowering caffeine, it's important to avoid high-fat meals with some bipolar medications. High-fat meals may delay the time it takes for some bipolar medications to take effect. Talk to your doctor about your medications and necessary dietary changes.

If you take MAO inhibitors (a certain class of antidepressant that includes Emsam, Nardil, and Parnate), it's important to avoid tyramine-containing foods. These foods can cause severe hypertension in people taking MAO inhibitors. Some foods high in tyramine are:

- Overly ripe bananas and banana peels
- Tap beer
- Fermented cheese
- Aged meats
- Some wines, such as Chianti
- Soy sauce in high quantities

Your doctor can give you a list of foods to avoid if you take these drugs. Also, avoid taking natural dietary supplements if you are taking bipolar medications. Supplements such as St. John's wort and SAM-e are touted to treat moderate depression. A few studies show benefit for some people with depression. But these natural therapies can interact with antidepressants and other bipolar medications. Discuss any natural dietary supplement with your doctor to make sure it is safe.

What About Alcohol and Bipolar Disorder?
Instructions for most psychiatric medications warn users not to drink alcohol, but people with bipolar disorder frequently abuse alcohol and other drugs. The abuse is possibly an attempt to self-medicate or to treat their disturbing mood symptoms, and they may also cause mood symptoms that can mimic those of bipolar disorder.

Alcohol is a depressant. That is why many people use it as a tranquilizer at the end of a hard day or as an assist for tense social situations. While some patients stop drinking when they are depressed, it is more common that someone with bipolar disorder drinks during low moods. According to research, people with bipolar disorder are five times more likely to develop alcohol misuse and dependence than the rest of the population.

The link between bipolar disorder and substance abuse is explosive. Alcohol is a leading trigger of depressive episodes in many people who are genetically vulnerable for depression or bipolar disorder. About 15% of all adults who have a psychiatric illness in any given year also experience a co-occurring substance abuse disorder. This disorder can seriously complicate treatment.

Drinking grapefruit juice while on Bipolar drugs

Be careful. Talk to your doctor or pharmacist about eating grapefruit or drinking grapefruit juice with your bipolar medication. Grapefruit juice may increase the blood levels of certain bipolar medications. This includes some anticonvulsants. Taking benzodiazepines -- Klonopin, Xanax, Valium, Ativan -- with grapefruit juice may cause excessive impairment and even toxicity.

Should I take Bipolar medication with or without food?

Each bipolar medication is different. So, talk with your doctor or pharmacist before taking the first dose. Some bipolar drugs can be taken with or without food. Others are less effective if taken with food. Your doctor or pharmacist will have the latest recommendations on taking the bipolar medication so you can safely take the medicine and get the full benefit of the drug.

In the next chapter we will be looking at rights in the workplace for those with bipolar disorder.

Now read the main points from Chapter 11 overleaf

****

Main points from Chapter 11

- Although there is no specific bipolar diet, nevertheless, it is very important indeed to make wise dietary choices that will help you maintain a healthy weight and stay well. This applies to all people, whether bi-polar sufferers or not.

- It is generally acknowledged that eating fatty fish at least two times a week is good for most people

- If you're a vegetarian or vegan looking for possible benefits of fish oil, go with nuts. Walnuts, flaxseed, and canola oil contain alpha-linolenic acid (ALA), which is converted to omega-3 fatty acid in the body.

- Some general dietary recommendations for treating bipolar disorder include getting only moderate amounts of caffeine and not stopping caffeine use abruptly, avoiding high-fat meals to lower the risk for obesity, watching your salt if you have high blood pressure but not skimping on salt if you are being prescribed lithium since low salt intake can cause higher levels of lithium in the blood and following your doctor's instructions to stay away from foods that may affect your specific bipolar medication, if any.

- Avoid taking natural dietary supplements if you are taking bipolar medications.

- The link between bipolar disorder and substance abuse is explosive. Alcohol is a leading trigger of depressive episodes in many people who are genetically vulnerable for depression or bipolar disorder.

****

Chapter 12

Rights in the Workplace for Those with Bipolar Disorder

Rights of the employee who has bipolar disorder
Alongside stress, mental health problems are now the leading cause of absence from work. However, taking sick leave is no longer considered the best solution-for employees or employers. The chances of individuals returning to work after a prolonged leave of absence are slim. In recent years, there has been a move away from sick leave to a more optimistic plan of work-based recovery.

Originally piloted in Wales and now rolled out throughout the UK, the governments fit-note programme sees work as a prescription towards recovery. The fit-note highlights areas of suitable employment in respect of an identified illness. The Fit note aims to encourage communication between doctor, patient and employer to help facilitate a return to work as soon as possible.

Working with bipolar
People with mental health problems generally experience prejudice, both in wider society and also in the workplace. This is

largely down to ignorance. An employer has a duty to provide a working environment that encourages good mental health. They also have a duty to combat any damaging practices within the workplace, such as bullying.

By educating staff about mental health, their preconceptions can be challenged.

Warning signs at work

Where you work and what you do will have an effect on you and will result in varying amounts of stress. As we have discussed earlier, stress is very much the enemy of a person suffering with bi-polar disorder. To maintain a healthy and productive working role it is important to feel that you have control over your work, as well as understanding the demands of your job.

The most common causes of work stress and mental health problems are increased work intensity, less security, less autonomy, target driven work cultures, which are increasing, and bullying and harassment. Look out for warning signs that your work is being affected by your condition. If you start to notice any of these warning signs then it is time to get some support. You need to talk to your manager or your HR department and they should work with you to make any changes needed. Avoiding the problem will make things worse, it is far better to deal with the issues sooner rather than later.

Examples of different warning signs

For those with bipolar, the following should alert you to the fact that something is wrong:

- Decreased concentration and memory
- Difficulties making a decision
- Nervousness and fear
- Sadness
- Headaches and chest pains
- Sleep disturbance and fatigue
- Being less agreeable with others
- Increased use of substances
- Repetitive thinking
- Negative thinking
- Frustration and irritability
- Weight fluctuation
- Taking risks with health.

Medication

There may be times when you have to change your medication following advice from your GP or psychiatrist. It is therefore important that your employer understands this and allows for periods of absence whilst you adjust.

Self-management

We discussed self-management earlier in the book. Self-management is about recognising triggers of an episode of mania or depression and managing your lifestyle around them to avoid them. Some of the most common triggers are sleep deprivation, relationship problems and, in some cases, a reaction to excess amounts of caffeine, alcohol or cigarettes. The majority of these problems can be avoided if managed properly. For situations outside your control, it is important that safety nets are in place to avoid illness. For example, being allowed time off to attend outpatient appointments or counselling an help head off an episode of manic depression.

Support

An employee with bipolar disorder has a responsibility to know their personal management needs and to inform their employer about their condition. Correspondingly, it is the employer's responsibility to recognise that the individual is attempting to manage their illness and to put simple policies in place to prevent unnecessary stress or anxiety for all their employees. There is a clear framework of law which covers bi-polar disorder: The Health and Safety at Work Act 1974, and the Equality Act 2010.

The Health and Safety at Work Act 1974

Under this Act, all employers have a duty of reasonable care for their employees. This includes the mental well-being of an individual. Employers must assess all health and safety risks, take preventative action and carry out health and safety training in the workplace. The responsibility for monitoring these acts rests with the Health and Safety Executive (HSE). The HSE, in addition to assisting the employer, can also serve notices and set deadlines to encourage development in areas of safety.

The Equality Act 2010
New ways of claiming disability discrimination have been introduced with the Equality Act. Direct discrimination and harassment based on association (an individual who is associated with a disabled person) or perception (an individual who looks as though they have a disability which they do not have) under the Equality Act is also unlawful.

The Equality Act 2010 sets out when someone is considered to be disabled and protected from discrimination. The definition is quite wide - so check it even if you don't think you're disabled. For example, you might be covered if you have a learning difficulty, dyslexia or autism. The Act also covers Bi-Polar.

The definition is set out in section 6 of the Equality Act 2010. It says you're disabled if:
- you have a physical or mental impairment
- that impairment has a substantial and long-term adverse effect on your ability to carry out normal day-to-day activities.

Some impairments are automatically treated as a disability. You'll be covered if you have:

- cancer, including skin growths that need removing before they become cancerous
- a visual impairment - this means you're certified as blind, severely sight impaired, sight impaired or partially sighted
- multiple sclerosis
- an HIV infection - even if you don't have any symptoms
- a severe, long-term disfigurement - for example severe facial scarring or a skin disease.

These are covered in Schedule 1, Part 1 of the Equality Act 2010 and in Regulation 7 of the Equality Act 2010 (Disability) Regulations 2010.

You have an 'impairment' if your physical or mental abilities are reduced in some way compared to most people. It could be the result of a medical condition - like arthritis in your hands that means you can't grip or carry things as well as other people.

Your impairment doesn't have to stop you doing anything, as long as it makes it harder. It might cause you pain, make things take much longer than they should or mean that you're unable to do an activity more than once.

Conditions which aren't impairments

Some conditions aren't disabilities under the Equality Act 2010. They include:
- hayfever

- tattoos or piercings
- voyeurism or exhibitionism
- a tendency to set fire to things
- a tendency to steal things
- a tendency to physically or sexually abuse others.

The full list is in the Equality Act 2010 (Disability) Regulations 2010.

Long-term impairment
A long-term effect means something that has affected you or is likely to affect you for at least a year. For example, if you had an operation that will make walking difficult for at least a year, that's long term.

Your impairment will still be considered to be long term if the effects are likely to come and go. These are known as 'fluctuating or recurring' effects. For example, you've had periods of depression for a few months at a time but then months in between where it doesn't affect you. Each episode of depression lasts less than 12 months, but it can meet the definition of long term if:
- it has a substantial adverse effect when it happens, and
- it could well happen again.

Your impairment will also still be considered to be long term if it's likely to affect you for the rest of your life even if that's going to be less than a year. The definition of what is long term is in Schedule 1 of the Equality Act 2010.

If your condition's getting worse
If you have a long-term condition that's getting worse, the effect on your day-to-day activities doesn't have to be substantial as long as it's likely to become substantial in the future. This is called a 'progressive condition'.

If you take medication or have treatment for your disability
The legal test is that you should look at the impact of your impairment without any medication or treatment. Treatment includes things like counselling as well as medication. For example, if you have arthritis and use a walking stick, think about how hard it would be for you to walk without it.

If you have a sight impairment which can be cured by wearing glasses or contact lenses, you'll need to think about how your day-to-day activities are affected when you're wearing them.

The Government has published a code of practice, under the DDA, to provide practical guidance about the elimination of discrimination against disabled people in the field of employment. A code does not impose legal obligations, but industrial tribunals and courts must take account of the code, where relevant, when considering cases.

Return to work

If you have been on sick leave, it is very useful to arrange a return-to-work meeting to discuss your needs and your employer's expectations. You might find it useful to include your psychiatrist in the meeting. if this can be arranged. You can also request union representation if this is available. During this meeting, you should discuss and agree any adjustments that need to be made. Agree how progress will be monitored and what colleagues will be told. You should ask your employer to identify specific tasks and roles for your return and confirm a suitable return date. It is very important that you believe that you are ready to go back and engage positively in the workplace.

Access to work

This is a Department of Work and Pensions scheme designed to financially assist employers with costs beyond that of reasonable adjustments, helping to produce a more efficient support system in the workplace. Examples can include awareness training for staff, sickness cover for those with a fluctuating condition and any specialist equipment to assist in adapting to roles. You must be in employment to qualify for access to work. You should visit www.direct.gov.uk for more details.

In the next chapter we will be looking at welfare benefits available to those with bipolar disorder.

Now read the main points from Chapter 12 overleaf.

Main points from Chapter 12

- Alongside stress, mental health problems are now the leading cause of absence from work. However, taking sick leave is no longer considered the best solution-for employees or employers.

- People with mental health problems generally experience prejudice, both in wider society and also in the workplace. This is largely down to ignorance. An employer has a duty to provide a working environment that encourages good mental health. They also have a duty to combat any damaging practices within the workplace, such as bullying. By educating staff about mental health, their preconceptions can be challenged.

- An employee with bipolar disorder has a responsibility to know their personal management needs and to inform their employer about their condition. Correspondingly, it is the employer's responsibility to recognise that the individual is attempting to manage their illness and to put simple policies in place to prevent unnecessary stress or anxiety for all their employees. There is a clear framework of law which covers bi-polar disorder: The Health and safety at Work Act 1974 and the Equality Act 2010.

****

Chapter 13

Welfare Benefits Available for those with Bipolar Disorder

The range of welfare benefits available

As someone with bipolar disorder, you will need to understand how the benefit system works and just what you may be entitled to if you are placed in a position where you are finding work difficult and you have to either work part time or give up work altogether.

The summary in appendix 1 covers the main benefits likely to impact on you:
- Universal Credit
- Employment and Support Allowance
- Severe Disablement Allowance
- Job seekers allowance
- Income Support (IS)
- Statutory Sick Pay (SSP)
- Disability Living Allowance (DLA) and Personal Independence Payment (PIP)
- Housing benefit

Checking your benefit entitlement

Although the aforementioned benefits cover the main benefits available there are a number of other benefits to which you may be entitled, depending on your circumstances. The Department for Work and Pensions (DWP) and your local council are not obliged to inform you which benefits you are entitled to, which means it is your responsibility to ensure you are claiming all of the relevant benefits.

If you are having problems with benefits then a welfare rights adviser may be able to help. This is someone that specialises in benefits. They can check that you are receiving everything you are entitled to, assist with claims and help with appeals if anything goes wrong. You can find a local adviser by contacting a local advice agency such as a Citizens Advice Bureau. If you have a support package as a bipolar sufferer then the person representing you will guide you towards an advisor.

Appendix 1 outlines all of the main benefits available. There are a number of organisations which give detailed and expert help where needed. They are:

Step change debt charity www.stepchange.org
Citizens advice www.citizensadvice.org.uk
Gov.uk-the various Gov.uk sites delaing with individual specific benefits. Detailed advice is available concerning all aspects of each benefit and how ro go about claiming.
Turn2us www.Turn2us.org.uk

Conclusion

Hopefully, this wide-ranging book has touched on most of the areas of concern of those who have bipolar disorder. At the beginning, we described bipolar generally and then throughout the book we discussed the many aspects of the disorder that need to be understood, such as support and medication, the role of the GP and psychiatric profession and also the benefits of cognitive behavioural therapy.

Areas such as the family and welfare benefits, plus the rights of the employee in the workplace have also been covered.

My own personal experience of bipolar disorder has been through friends and I have seen at first-hand how this can affect people's lives and lead to a downward spiral. I have suffered with those people.

The outcome of my experience is this book, which I sincerely hope will go a long way to promoting an understanding of the condition and also help the reader raise his or her awareness of what they can do to alleviate the problems associated with bipolar.

Doreen Jarrett.
2024

Useful addresses and Websites

Care Quality Commission (CQC)-London Office
167-169 Great Portland Street
London
W1W 5PF
Tel: 020 7274 3116

National Association of Citizens Advice Bureau
www.citizensadvice.org.uk
Through the main site you can get advice concerning law in England, Ireland, Scotland and Wales.

Department for Work and Pensions
www.gov.uk/government/organisations/department-for-work-pensions

Depression Alliance (now part of MIND)
www.mind.org.uk

Mental Health Foundation: UK London Office
Studio 2
197 Long Lane
London SE1 4PD
Tel:020 7803 1100
www.mentalhealth.org.uk

MIND (The National Association for Mental Health)
Tel: 0300 123 3393
www.mind.org.uk

Mood Swings Network
36 New Mount Street
Manchester M4 4DE
Tel: 0161 832 3736
www.moodswings.org.uk

Bipolar UK National Office
0333 323 3880
www.bipolaruk.org.uk

Bi-polar UK has the most extensive range of resources to aid and assist all who need help and information in this area.

The Scottish Association for Mental Health
www.samh.org.uk

The Northern Ireland Association for Mental Health
www.communityni

Self-help websites for bipolar & depression
www.bipolarworld.net

An American information and support site for people with bipolar disorder, run mainly by service users. Includes chat rooms and internet-search service for bipolar-related topics.

www.mcmanweb.com

An American site run by someone with a diagnosis of bipolar disorder, who previously worked as a financial journalist. It provides information and updates on clinical research into bipolar disorder, as well as input from other service users and a discussion forum.

www.mentalhealth.org.uk

This Mental Health Foundation website covers mental-health issues relating to children and adults. It also funds research into these areas and provides information on this. A number of the initiatives being developed by the Mental Health Foundation are described here, including their development of services with a significant amount of user involvement.

www.mind.org.uk

The British site for MIND. A broad-ranging site covering self-help information, information on local MIND groups and email contacts. This site also provides information on current MIND campaigns and projects and opportunities within the organisation for voluntary and paid employment.

www.pendulum.org
A site providing information on recent developments in bipolar disorder. Books relevant to bipolar disorder are listed and recent, usually American, research is highlighted. Informal jokes – and fun-pages are included. The site has a bipolar-focused search engine.

Bipolar and Pregnancy
Action on Postpartum Psychosis (APP) www.app-network.org is a charity run by a group of women who have suffered with this illness, clinicians and academic researchers. They have a website to provide support and information for other women in a similar position and their partners: www.app-network.org

APP would also be interested to hear from women with bipolar who are pregnant or considering pregnancy, so they can keep them informed of research projects which might interest them. You can join for free and receive occasional emails about the latest news and research. The website also contains advice on recovery, personal stories and details of a Peer Support Network using trained volunteers who have recovered from postpartum psychosis themselves.

As discussed above, Bipolar UK the national charity for people affected by bipolar including families, carers and loved ones. They provide a range of services across England and Wales including self-help groups and regularly run workshops at their

Annual Conference on the issues facing women who have bipolar and want to start a family. www.bipolaruk.org.uk

There is also a thread on the charity's web-based forum – the eCommunity – accessed via the website, where these issues are discussed and women can support each other.

Other useful websites:

The Royal College of Psychiatrists (www.rcpsych.ac.uk)
This site has excellent leaflets on postnatal depression and postpartum psychosis.

Postpartum Support International – PSI (www.postpartum.net)
An international network that links volunteers, support groups, and professionals, particularly strong in the US.

PNI ORG UK (Post Natal Illness) (www.pni.org.uk)
An information site for sufferers and survivors of all types of postnatal illness.

Bipolar Disorder Research Network (www.bdrn.org)
BDRN is a group of researchers and research participants in the UK undertaking a major study investigating the underlying causes of bipolar disorder.

*

Cry-sis (www.cry-sis.org.uk)-Helpline: 0800 448 0737. Provides self-help and support for families with excessively crying and sleepless and demanding babies.

Family Action (www.family-action.org.uk)
Tel: 0808 802 6666. Support and practical help for families affected by mental illness, including 'Newpin' services – offering support to parents of children under-5 whose mental health is affecting their ability to provide safe parenting.

Home Start (www.home-start.org.uk)
Tel: 0116 464 5490 (England) 07747 487 938 (Northern Ireland) 0131 281 0879 (Scotland) 0292 0491181 (Wales). Support and practical help for families with at least one child under-5.

Help offered to parents finding it hard to cope for many reasons. These include PND or other mental illness, isolation, bereavement, illness of parent or child.

Netmums (www.netmums.com/pnd)
Parenting Support. A website offering support and information on pregnancy and parenting. There is also information on local resources and support groups.

The Samaritans (www.samaritans.org)
24-hour helpline 116 123   email: jo@ samaritans.org

Index

Access to work, 108
Aggressive behaviour, 7
Aggressiveness, 76
Amitriptyline, 34
Anger, 70, 71, 73
Anticonvulsant drugs, 33
Anti-depressants, 34
Anti-parkinsonian drugs, 36
Antipsychotic drugs, 36
Appetit, 8
Assertiveness, 3, 74, 75

Behavioural therapy, 52
Bipolar 1 disorder, 9
Bipolar 2 disorder, 9
Breathing Exercise, 66

Caffeine, 81, 95
Carbamazepine, 33
Care co-ordinators, 47
Care Programme Approach (CPA), 44
Child and Adolescent Mental Health Service (CAMHS), 40, 49
Childhood bi-polar disorder, 11
Childhood distress, 11
Cognitive behavioral therapy, 45
Cognitive therapy, 52
Community mental health teams, 44
Community psychiatric nurse, 45
Cyclothymia, 9

Delayed sleep phase syndrome, 79
Delusions, 5
Department for Work and Pensions (DWP, 111
Depression, 6, 7, 10, 60, 113
Diet, 25, 92
Dietary supplements, 96
Disability Living Allowance (DLA, 110

Equality Act 2010, 103, 104, 109

Family Issues, 3, 86
Family therapy, 46
Fatigue, 8
Fish Oil, 93

Grapefruit Juice, 97
Grief, 11, 87, 91
Group therapy, 46

Health and Safety at Work Act 1974, 103
Hospitalization, 47
Hypomania, 6, 7

Income Support, 110
Income Support (IS), 110
Insomnia, 79
Irregular sleep-wake schedules, 79
Irritability, 8

Job seekers allowance, 110

Lamotrigine, 33
Largacti, 36
Lithium, 31, 32
Lithium carbonate, 32
Lithium Citrate, 32

Managing bipolar disorder, 19
Manic episodes, 6
Medication, 3, 29, 31, 97, 102
Minor tranquillisers, 37
Mixed episodes, 6

National Institute for Health and Care Excellence (NICE, 29, 39
Neuroleptics, 36
Non-Assertiveness, 74

Omega 3, 25

Parental support, 86
Parkinson's, 10, 18
Personal Independence Payment (PIP), 110
Pregnancy, 14, 116
Progressive Muscle Relaxation, 67
Prozac, 35
Psychodynamic therapists, 46
Psychoeducation, 45
Psychotherapy, 45

Relaxation, 25, 65, 67
Relaxation techniques, 25
REM (rapid eye movement, 79, 85
Return to work, 108
Rights in the Workplace, 100
Risky behaviour, 7

Sadness, 102
Self-management, 102
Seroxat, 35
Shame, 3, 58
Sleep disturbance, 11, 102
Sodium valproate, 33
Spouses, 87, 91
Statutory Sick Pay (SSP), 110, 121, 124
Stigma, 3, 58, 59
Stigmatisation, 58, 63
Stress, 21, 24, 65, 73, 82
Suicide, 8
Suppressing Anger, 71

Trcyclic anti-depressants, 34

Vicious cycles, 64, 65, 73
Visualization, 68

Weight fluctuation, 102
Welfare benefits, 110
Working with bipolar, 100

****

Appendix 1

A Comprehensive Guide to Welfare Benefits available in the 2024/2025 tax year.

This brief guide will help to shed light on the range of benefits available to bi-polar sufferers and families. The following benefits are covered:

	p
Universal Credit	123
Statutory Sick Pay (SSP)	126
Personal Independence Payment	126
Disability living allowance	137
Employment and Support allowance	147
Budgeting loans	150
Job seekers allowance	151
Income Support	161
Housing benefit	164
Council tax reduction	173
The range of other benefits available	174

Universal Credit

Although below we discuss the wide range of benefits available it should be noted that Universal Credit has replaced the below benefits for most people:

- Housing Benefit
- income-related Employment and Support Allowance (ESA)
- income-based Jobseeker's Allowance (JSA)

- Child Tax Credit
- Working Tax Credit
- Income Support

You might be able to get Universal Credit if you're not working or you're on a low income. Universal Credit works differently from the old benefits - so it's important to know the differences. The biggest differences are:

- you can get Universal Credit if you're unemployed but also if you're working
- you'll usually get a single payment each month, rather than weekly or fortnightly
- instead of getting separate housing benefit, your rent will usually be paid directly to you as part of your monthly Universal Credit payment.

How Universal Credit works

You'll usually get one monthly payment to cover your living costs. If you claim Universal Credit as a couple, you and your partner will get one payment between the 2 of you. The payment is made up of a basic 'standard allowance' and extra payments that might apply to you depending on your circumstances.

You might be able to get extra payments if you:
- look after one or more children

- work and pay for childcare
- need help with housing costs
- are disabled or have a health condition
- are a carer for a disabled person or you have a disabled child

If you get help with rent
If your UC payment includes help with rent (see below Housing Benefit) you'll usually need to pay your landlord each month even if you live in social housing. You can ask the DWP to pay your rent directly to your landlord if you're in debt, have rent arrears or are struggling with money.

If you're working
You can work and still get Universal Credit - your Universal Credit will reduce gradually as you earn more. Your Universal Credit will go up if your job ends or you earn less.

If you're self-employed, your payment might also be affected by how much the DWP expect you to earn each month - this expected amount is called your 'minimum income floor'..

Claiming other benefits if you get Universal Credit
You should apply for Council Tax Reduction - if you get it, it won't reduce the amount of Universal Credit you get. If you're disabled, you should check if you're eligible for Personal Independence Payment (PIP). If you're responsible for a disabled

child, you should check if you can claim Disability Living Allowance (DLA) for your child. Getting PIP or DLA won't reduce the amount of Universal Credit you get.

You can also claim other benefits if you have enough national insurance contributions. For example:
- if you're unemployed, , also called 'new style' JSA
- if you can't work because of illness or disability.

Statutory Sick Pay (SSP)

SSP is not a really a welfare benefit. It is paid by employers to employees who are unable to work due to sickness. Employers are under a legal obligation to pay SSP for a maximum of 28 weeks if you meet the criteria. Although there is a standard rate of SSP some employers will pay more. This is called contractual sick pay. You should check your contract of employment to see what you will be paid in the event of sickness. When your SSP is due to end, your employer will send you a form called an SSP1. If you are still too unwell to work at the point when SSP stops, you should claim ESA.

Personal Independence Payment

What PIP is for
Personal Independence Payment (PIP) can help with extra living costs if you have both:
- a long-term physical or mental health condition or disability
- difficulty doing certain everyday tasks or getting around because of your condition.

You can get PIP even if you're working, have savings or are getting most other benefits.

How PIP works
There are 2 parts to PIP:
- a daily living part - if you need help with everyday tasks
- a mobility part - if you need help with getting around.

Whether you get one or both parts and how much you get depends on how difficult you find everyday tasks and getting around. If you might have less than 12 months to live, you'll automatically get the daily living part. Whether you get the mobility part depends on your needs. Find out how to claim and how much you'll get if you might have 12 months or less to live.

Daily living part
You might get the daily living part of PIP if you need help with:
- preparing food
- eating and drinking
- managing your medicines or treatments
- washing and bathing
- using the toilet
- dressing and undressing
- reading
- managing your money
- socialising and being around other people
- talking, listening and understanding.

Mobility part

You might get the mobility part of PIP if you need help with:
- working out a route and following it
- physically moving around
- leaving your home

You do not have to have a physical disability to get the mobility part. You might also be eligible if you have difficulty getting around because of a cognitive or mental health condition, like anxiety.

How difficulty with tasks is assessed

The Department for Work and Pensions (DWP) will assess how difficult you find daily living and mobility tasks. For each task they'll look at:
- whether you can do it safely
- how long it takes you
- how often your condition affects this activity
- whether you need help to do it, from a person or using extra equipment.

Your carer could get Carer's Allowance if you have substantial caring needs.

Help with PIP

If you need help understanding or applying for PIP you can:
- get help from Citizens Advice
- watch PIP video guides with British Sign Language
- use easy read guides which explain PIP

If you live in Scotland

You need to apply for Adult Disability Payment (ADP) instead of PIP. If you currently get PIP, you'll be automatically moved to ADP by summer 2024. When the move begins, you'll get letters from DWP and Social Security Scotland. Read more about the moving process.

If you move from Scotland to England or Wales

If you get ADP and move from Scotland to England or Wales, you must make a new claim for PIP instead.

Your ADP will stop 13 weeks after you move – apply for PIP as soon as possible after moving or your payments could be affected.

If you get Disability Living Allowance (DLA)

Disability Living Allowance (DLA) is being replaced by PIP for most adults. You'll keep getting DLA if:

- you're under 16
- you were born on or before 8 April 1948.

If you were born after 8 April 1948, DWP will invite you to apply for PIP. You do not need to do anything until DWP writes to you about your DLA unless your circumstances change. You can get Personal Independence Payment (PIP) if all of the following apply to you:

- you're 16 or over
- you have a long-term physical or mental health condition or disability
- you have difficulty doing certain everyday tasks or getting around
- you expect the difficulties to last for at least 12 months from when they started.

You must also be under State Pension age if you've not received PIP before.

If you live in Scotland, you need to apply for Adult Disability Payment (ADP) instead. If you're over State Pension age, you can apply for Attendance Allowance instead. Or if you've received PIP before, you can still make a new claim if you were eligible for it in the year before you reached State Pension age.

If you get other benefits or income

You can get PIP at the same time as all other benefits, except Armed Forces Independence Payment. If you get Constant Attendance Allowance you'll get less of the daily living part of PIP. If you get War Pensioners' Mobility Supplement you will not get the mobility part of PIP. You can get PIP if you're working or have savings.

If you've recently returned from living abroad

To apply for PIP, you usually need to:
- have lived in England, Scotland or Wales for at least 2 of the last 3 years
- be living in one of these countries when you apply.

If you've recently returned from living in the EU, Switzerland, Norway, Iceland or Liechtenstein, you might be able to get PIP sooner.

If you live abroad

You might still be able to get PIP if you either:
- live in the EU, Switzerland, Norway, Iceland or Liechtenstein - you can only get help with daily living tasks

- work in the Armed Forces or are a family member of someone who does.

If you're not a British citizen

You must:

- normally live in or show that you intend to settle in the UK, Ireland, the Isle of Man or the Channel Islands
- not be subject to immigration control (unless you're a sponsored immigrant)

If you're from the EU, Switzerland, Norway, Iceland or Liechtenstein, you and your family usually also need settled or pre-settled status under the EU Settlement Scheme to get PIP. The deadline to apply to the scheme was 30 June 2021 for most people, but you might still be able to apply. Check if you can still apply to the EU Settlement Scheme. You might still be able to get PIP if you're a refugee or have humanitarian protection status.

How much you'll get

How much Personal Independence Payment (PIP) you get depends on how difficult you find:

- everyday activities ('daily living' tasks)
- getting around ('mobility' tasks)

PIP amounts

	Lower weekly rate	Higher weekly rate
Daily living part	£72.65	£108.55

	Lower weekly rate	Higher weekly rate
Mobility part	£28.70	£75.75

PIP is tax free. The amount you get is not affected by your income or savings. Tell the Department for Work and Pensions (DWP) straight away if there's a change in your personal circumstances or how your condition affects you.

How you're paid

PIP is usually paid every 4 weeks.

Your decision letter tells you:
- the date of your first payment
- what day of the week you'll usually be paid
- how long you'll get PIP for
- when and if your claim will be reviewed.

If your payment date is on a bank holiday, you'll usually be paid before the bank holiday. After that you'll continue to get paid as normal. All benefits, pensions and allowances are paid into your bank, building society or credit union account.

Other help you can get

If you get the mobility part of PIP, you might be eligible for a:
- Blue Badge
- vehicle tax discount or exemption
- Motability Scheme vehicle, if you get the higher mobility rate of PIP.

If you get either the daily living or mobility part of PIP you're eligible for a Disabled Persons Railcard. You may be able to get a discount on Council Tax and local bus travel. Contact your local council to check. If someone helps to care for you, they may be able to get Carer's Allowance or Carer's Credit.

If you get other benefits and PIP
You may get a top-up (called a disability premium) if you get:
- Income Support
- income-based Jobseeker's Allowance (JSA)
- income-related Employment and Support Allowance (ESA)
- Housing Benefit.

You might get the disability element of Working Tax Credit if you're eligible. If you get Constant Attendance Allowance you'll get less of the daily living part of PIP. If you get War Pensioners' Mobility Supplement you will not get the mobility part of PIP.

How to claim
Before you apply for Personal Independence Payment (PIP), check if you're eligible. If you live in Scotland, you need to apply for Adult Disability Payment (ADP) instead.

Start your claim by phone
You need to:
- Call the 'PIP new claims' phone line. You'll then be sent a form that asks about your condition.
- Complete and return the form. The address is on the form.

- You might need to have an assessment, if more information is needed.

There's a different way to claim if you might have 12 months or less to live.

If you need someone to help you

You can:

- ask for them to be added to your call - you cannot do this if you use textphone
- ask someone else to call on your behalf - you'll need to be with them when they call.

Before you start

You'll need:

- your contact details, for example telephone number
- your date of birth
- your National Insurance number, if you have one (you can find this on letters about tax, pensions and benefits)
- your bank or building society account number and sort code
- your doctor or health worker's name, address and telephone number
- dates and addresses for any time you've spent in a care home or hospital
- dates for any time you spent abroad for more than 4 weeks at a time, and the countries you visited.

PIP new claims phone line

Telephone: 0800 917 2222

Textphone: 0800 917 7777

Relay UK (if you cannot hear or speak on the phone): 18001 then 0800 917 2222

British Sign Language (BSL) video relay service if you're on a computer - find out how to use the service on mobile or tablet
Calling from abroad: +44 191 218 7766

Monday to Friday, 8am to 5pm

Start your claim by post
You can start a claim by post instead, but it takes longer to get a decision. Send a letter to 'Personal Independence Payment New Claims'. You'll be sent a form asking for your personal information, such as your address and your age. Fill in and return the form. You'll then be sent a form which asks about your disability or condition.

Personal Independence Payment New Claims
Post Handling Site B
Wolverhampton
WV99 1AH

Completing and returning the form about your condition
If you apply by phone or post, you'll usually get a form called 'How your disability affects you' within 2 weeks. Fill in the form using the guidance that comes with it and return it to the address on the form. Include supporting documents if you have them - for example, prescription lists, care plans, or information from your doctor or others involved in your care. You have 1 month to return it. Contact the PIP enquiry line if you need more time or have questions.

Apply online

You can only apply for PIP online in some areas. You'll need to check your postcode when you start your application. To start your claim online you'll need your:

- National Insurance number
- email address
- mobile phone.

Apply now

If you've already registered, you can sign in to your PIP account.

If you need to have an assessment

You'll be invited to an assessment with a health professional if more information is needed. They'll ask about:

- how your condition affects your daily living and mobility tasks
- any treatments you've had or will have.

They might ask you to do some simple movements to show how you manage some activities. The assessment can be in person, over the phone or by video call. It usually takes 1 hour. If your assessment is in person, your invitation letter will explain how to attend your appointment safely.

Getting a decision

You'll get a letter that tells you whether you'll get PIP and the date of your first payment.

If you disagree with a decision

You can challenge a decision about your claim. This is called asking for 'mandatory reconsideration'.

Disability living allowance-Overview

Disability Living Allowance (DLA) is being replaced by other benefits. If you already get DLA, your claim might end. You'll get a letter telling you when this will happen and how you can apply for PIP or Adult Disability Payment.

If you're under 16

You can only apply for DLA if you're under 16 and you live in England or Wales. If you live in Scotland, you can apply for Child Disability Payment.

If you're over 16

You cannot apply for DLA. You can apply for:
- Personal Independence Payment (PIP) if you live in England or Wales and have not reached State Pension age
- Adult Disability Payment if you live in Scotland and have not reached State Pension age
- Attendance Allowance if you're State Pension age or older and do not get DLA.

If you already get DLA

If you were born on or before 8 April 1948, you'll continue to get DLA as long as you're eligible for it. If you were born after 8 April 1948, your DLA will end. You'll get a letter telling you when that will happen. You'll continue to get DLA until that date. Unless your circumstances change, you do not need to do anything until you get this letter. If you live in Scotland, you can choose to move from DLA to Adult Disability Payment before your DLA claim ends by contacting the Disability Service Centre.

If your DLA claim is ending-If you live in England or Wales

If your DLA is ending, you'll get a letter inviting you to apply for Personal Independence Payment (PIP). If you do apply, you'll need to do it within 28 days. DLA will continue to be paid until at least 28 days after a decision is made about your PIP application. If you're eligible for PIP, you'll start getting PIP payments as soon as your DLA payments end.

If you live in Scotland

If your DLA is ending, you'll get letters telling you that you're being moved from DLA to Adult Disability Payment. You'll have no gaps in your payments. After you've moved over, Social Security Scotland will review what you should get from Adult Disability Payment based on your current circumstances.

Change of circumstances

You must contact the Disability Service Centre if your circumstances change, as this may affect how much DLA you get. For example:

- the level of help you need or your condition changes
- you go into hospital or a care home for more than 4 weeks
- a medical professional has said you might have 12 months or less to live
- you plan to go abroad for more than 4 weeks
- you're imprisoned or held in detention.

You must also contact the centre if:
- you change your name, address or bank details
- you want to stop receiving your benefit
- your doctor's details change.

You may be asked to claim Personal Independence Payment (PIP) or be told you're being moved from DLA to Adult Disability Payment after you report a change to your circumstances.

If you've been paid too much

You may have to repay the money if you:
- did not report a change straight away
- gave wrong information
- were overpaid by mistake.

If you disagree with a decision

You can challenge a decision about your DLA claim. This is called asking for 'mandatory reconsideration'.

DLA rates

You can no longer apply for DLA. Check what other benefits you could apply for. DLA is made up of 2 components (parts), the 'care component' and the 'mobility component'. To get DLA you must be eligible for at least one of the components. How much DLA you get depends on how your disability or health condition affects you.

If you need help looking after yourself

You might get the care component of DLA if you:
- need help with things like washing, dressing, eating, using the toilet or communicating your needs.

- need supervision to avoid putting yourself or others in danger
- need someone with you when you're on dialysis
- cannot prepare a cooked main meal.

You can get this part if no one is actually giving you the care you need, or you live alone.

Care component	Weekly rate	Level of help you need
Lowest	£28.70	Help for some of the day or with preparing cooked meals
Middle	£72.65	Frequent help or constant supervision during the day, supervision at night or someone to help you while on dialysis
Highest	£108.55	Help or supervision throughout both day and night, or a medical professional has said you might have 12 months or less to live

If you get DLA and Constant Attendance Allowance, the care component of your DLA will be reduced by the amount of Constant Attendance Allowance you get.

If you have walking difficulties

You might get the mobility component of DLA if, when using your normal aid, you:
- cannot walk
- can only walk a short distance without severe discomfort
- could become very ill if you try to walk.

You might also get it if you:
- have no feet or legs
- are assessed as 100% blind and at least 80% deaf and you need someone with you when outdoors
- are severely mentally impaired with severe behavioural problems and get the highest rate of care for DLA
- need supervision most of the time when walking outdoors
- are certified as severely sight impaired and you were aged between 3 and 64 on 11 April 2011

Mobility component	Weekly rate	Level of help you need
Lower	£28.70	Guidance or supervision outdoors
Higher	£75.75	You have any other, more severe, walking difficulty

You must contact the Disability Service Centre if your circumstances change, for example your condition improves or you need more help.

Assessments

You might get a letter saying you need to attend an assessment to check the level of help you need. The letter explains why, and where you must go. Your benefit may be stopped if you do not go. At the assessment, you'll be asked for identification. You can use a passport or any 3 of the following:
- birth certificate
- a full driving licence
- life assurance policy
- bank statements.

How you're paid

DLA is usually paid every 4 weeks on a Wednesday. If your payment date is on a bank holiday, you will usually be paid before the bank holiday. After that you'll continue to get paid as normal. All benefits, pensions and allowances are paid into your bank or building society account.

Extra help

You could get extra benefits if you get Disability Living Allowance - check with the Disability Service Centre or the office dealing with your benefit. If your disability or health condition stops you from working and you're eligible for Universal Credit, you could get an extra amount on top of your Universal Credit standard allowance. If you get DLA and you work, you might also be able to get the disability element of Working Tax Credit (up to £3,935 a year, or up to £5,640 if your disability is severe). Contact HM Revenue and Customs (HMRC) to find out.

DLA for children

Overview

Disability Living Allowance (DLA) for children may help with the extra costs of looking after a child who:
- is under 16
- has difficulties walking or needs much more looking after than a child of the same age who does not have a disability.

They will need to meet all the eligibility requirements. The DLA rate is between £28.70 and £184.30 a week and depends on the level of help the child needs. This guide is also available in Welsh (Cymraeg), British Sign Language (BSL) and easy read format.

If your child lives in Scotland

You need to apply for Child Disability Payment instead of DLA for children. If your child is getting DLA for children but they have moved to Scotland, you'll need to report this change so they can get Child Disability Payment instead.

If your child moves from Scotland to England or Wales

If your child gets Child Disability Payment, you must:
- report this to Social Security Scotland
- make a new claim for DLA for children.

DLA rates for children

Disability Living Allowance (DLA) for children is a tax-free benefit made up of 2 components (parts). The child might qualify for one or both components.

Care component	Weekly rate
Lowest	£28.70
Middle	£72.65
Highest	£108.55
Mobility component	Weekly rate
Lower	£28.70
Higher	£75.75

Extra help

You might qualify for Carer's Allowance if you spend at least 35 hours a week caring for a child who gets the middle or highest care rate of DLA.

Eligibility

Usually, to qualify for Disability Living Allowance (DLA) for children the child must:

- be under 16 - anyone over 16 must apply for Personal Independence Payment (PIP)
- need extra looking after or have walking difficulties
- be in England, Wales, a European Economic Area (EEA) country or Switzerland when you claim - there are some exceptions, such as family members of the Armed Forces
- have lived in Great Britain for at least 6 of the last 12 months, if over 3 years old
- be habitually resident in the UK, Ireland, Isle of Man or the Channel Islands
- not be subject to immigration control.

If you're not a British citizen

If you and your child are from the EU, Switzerland, Norway, Iceland, or Liechtenstein, you will usually also need settled or pre-settled status under the EU Settlement Scheme to claim DLA for your child. The deadline to apply to the scheme was 30 June 2021 for most people, but you might still be able to apply. Check if you can still apply to the EU Settlement Scheme.

Children under 3

A child under 6 months must have lived in Great Britain for at least 13 weeks. A child aged between 6 months and 3 years must have lived in Great Britain for at least 26 of the last 156 weeks. The rules on residence do not normally apply if a medical professional has said the child might have 12 months or less to live.

The child's disability or health condition

The child's disability or health condition must mean at least one of the following apply:
- they need much more looking after than a child of the same age who does not have a disability
- they have difficulty getting about.

They must have had these difficulties for at least 3 months and expect them to last for at least 6 months. If a medical professional has said they might have 12 months or less to live, they do not need to have had these difficulties for 3 months.

Care component

The rate the child gets depends on the level of looking after they need, for example:
- lowest rate - help for some of the day
- middle rate - frequent help or constant supervision during the day, supervision at night or someone to help while they're on dialysis
- highest rate - help or supervision throughout both day and night, or a medical professional has said they might have 12 months or less to live.

Mobility component

The rate the child gets depends on the level of help they need getting about, for example:

- lowest rate - they can walk but need help and or supervision when outdoors
- highest rate - they cannot walk, can only walk a short distance without severe discomfort, could become very ill if they try to walk or they're blind or severely sight impaired.

There are also age limits to receiving the mobility component:

- lowest rate - the child must be 5 years or over
- highest rate - the child must be 3 years or over.

If your child is under these ages and you claim DLA for them, you should be sent a claim pack 6 months before they turn 3 and 6 months before they turn 5. You can then apply for the mobility component if you think they're eligible for it. If you have not received any claim packs and you think your child may be entitled to the mobility component, contact the Disability Service Centre

Employment Support Allowance-Overview

You can apply for Employment and Support Allowance (ESA) if you have a disability or health condition that affects how much you can work. ESA gives you:

- money to help with living costs if you're unable to work
- support to get back into work if you're able to.

You can apply if you're employed, self-employed or unemployed.

Eligibility

You can apply for New Style Employment and Support Allowance (ESA) if you're under State Pension age and you have a disability or health condition that affects how much you can work. You also need to have both:

- worked as an employee or have been self-employed
- paid enough National Insurance contributions, usually in the last 2 to 3 years - National Insurance credits also count.

You cannot get New Style ESA if you claim Jobseeker's Allowance (JSA) or Statutory Sick Pay

Claiming Universal Credit and New Style ESA

You might be able to get Universal Credit at the same time or instead of New Style ESA. If you get both benefits, your Universal Credit payment is reduced by the amount you get for New Style ESA. Your New Style ESA will usually be paid more regularly than Universal Credit. You'll also get different National Insurance credits which count towards your State Pension and help you qualify for other benefits.

If your Statutory Sick Pay (SSP) is due to end

You can apply for New Style ESA up to 3 months before your SSP ends. You'll start getting New Style ESA as soon as your SSP ends.

If you're working

You can apply whether you're in or out of work. There are conditions to working while claiming ESA.

What you'll get

How much you get will depend on what stage your application is at, as well as things like your age and whether you're able to get back into work. If you get New Style ESA you'll earn Class 1 National Insurance credits, which can help towards your State Pension and some benefits in the future.

What might affect how much you get paid

If you get New Style ESA

Your payments will be affected if you get more than £85 a week from a private pension. If you do, half of your private pension income over £85 will be subtracted from your ESA payments each week.

For example, if you get £100 a week from a private pension, then £7.50 will be subtracted from your ESA payment each week. If your private pension income is high enough, you could get no ESA payments. You would still get Class 1 National Insurance credits.

If you get income-related ESA

You cannot make a new claim for income-related ESA. You'll continue to get payments while you're eligible until your claim ends.

Your household income and savings worth £6,000 or more may affect how much you can get.

While your claim is being assessed

You'll normally get the 'assessment rate' for 13 weeks while your claim is being assessed.

This will be:

- up to £71.70 a week if you're aged under 25 (2024/25)
- up to £90.50 a week if you're aged 25 or over.

If it takes longer than 13 weeks to assess your claim, you'll continue getting the 'assessment rate' until you get a decision or until your ESA is due to end. Your ESA will be backdated if you're owed any money after 13 weeks.

After you're assessed
You'll be placed into one of 2 groups if you're entitled to ESA. If you're able to get back into work in the future, you'll be put into the work-related activity group. Otherwise, you'll be put into the support group. At 2024/5, you'll get:
- up to £90.50 a week if you're in the work-related activity group
- up to £138.20 a week if you're in the support group.

If you're in the support group
If you're in the support group and on income-related ESA, you're also entitled to the enhanced disability premium. You may also qualify for the severe disability premium.

How and when you're paid
You'll get paid ESA every 2 weeks.

Other benefits you can claim
You could get Universal Credit at the same time or instead of New Style ESA. The benefit cap may affect the total amount of benefit you can get. The cap will not affect you if you're in the support group.

If you're moving to Universal Credit from income-related ESA

If your income-related ESA claim is ending because you're making a new claim for Universal Credit, you'll automatically continue to get the amount of ESA you currently receive, as long as you're still eligible. You'll normally get this for 2 weeks, starting from the date of your new claim. The Department for Work and Pensions (DWP) will write to you telling you how this works. You do not need to pay this money back, and it will not affect the amount of Universal Credit you get.

Budgeting Loan

You can apply for a Budgeting Loan if you've been on income-related ESA for at least 6 months.

Working while you claim

You can usually work while you are claiming ESA if both of the following apply:
- you work less than 16 hours a week
- you do not earn more than £183.50 a week.

You can do as many hours of voluntary work as you like.

Job Seekers Allowance-How it works

You can apply for New Style Jobseeker's Allowance (JSA) to help you when you're looking for work. You cannot apply for income based JSA any more. If you're currently getting income based JSA, you'll keep getting payments while you're eligible until your claim ends. You could get Universal Credit at the same time or instead of New Style JSA. Check if you're eligible for Universal Credit.

What you need to do
- Check you're eligible.
- Make a claim for New Style Jobseeker's Allowance (JSA) and go to an interview at your local Jobcentre Plus office.
- Keep to your agreement to look for work. This agreement is called a 'Claimant Commitment' and you will create it at your interview.

Your JSA payments will be reduced or stopped if you do not keep to your agreement to look for work and cannot give a good reason.

What you'll get
There's a maximum amount you can get - but how much you're entitled to depends on your age.

Age	JSA weekly amount
Up to 24	up to £71.70
25 or over	up to £90.50

If you're moving to Universal Credit from income-based JSA
If your income-based JSA claim is ending because you're making a new claim for Universal Credit, you'll automatically continue to get the amount of JSA you currently receive, as long as you're still eligible. You'll normally get this for 2 weeks, starting from the date of your new claim. The Department for Work and Pensions (DWP) will write to you telling you how this works. You do not need to pay this money back, and it will not affect the amount of Universal Credit you get.

To be eligible for New Style Jobseeker's Allowance (JSA) you'll need to have both:
- worked as an employee
- paid Class 1 National Insurance contributions, usually in the last 2 to 3 years (National Insurance credits can also count)

You will not be eligible if you were self-employed and only paid Class 2 National Insurance contributions, unless you were working as a share fisherman or a volunteer development worker. You'll also need to:
- be 18 or over (there are some exceptions if you're 16 or 17 - contact Jobcentre Plus for advice)
- be under the State Pension age
- not be in full-time education
- be available for work
- not be working at the moment, or be working less than 16 hours per week on average
- not have an illness or disability which stops you from working
- live in the UK.

While you receive JSA, you'll need to take reasonable steps to look for work as agreed with your work coach. Your savings and your partner's income and savings will not affect your claim. You can get New Style Jobseeker's Allowance (JSA) for up to 182 days (about 6 months). After this you can talk to your work coach about your options.

Claiming Universal Credit and New Style JSA
You might be able to get Universal Credit at the same time or instead of New Style JSA. If you get both benefits, your New Style JSA payments:

- count as income when claiming Universal Credit
- will reduce the amount of Universal Credit you receive.

Your New Style JSA will usually be paid more regularly than Universal Credit. You'll also get different National Insurance credits which count towards your State Pension and help you qualify for other benefits. To apply, you'll need your:
- National Insurance number
- bank or building society account details (or those of a family member or trusted friend)
- employment details for the past 6 months, including employer contact details and dates you worked with them.

You'll also need to provide a statement letter if you receive any money from:
- your private pension
- your workplace pension
- an annuity you've bought.

To reclaim you need to apply again, even if your details have not changed. You can backdate your claim by up to 3 months in certain circumstances.

Apply online
You cannot apply online if you're under 18 or if you're applying as an appointee on someone else's behalf.

If you cannot apply online or need alternative formats
You can apply another way if any of the following apply:
- you're aged 16 to 17

- you're applying as an appointee on someone else's behalf
- you need help applying
- you need communications to be sent to you in an alternative format, such as braille, large print or audio CD.

You need to either:
- contact Jobcentre Plus if you live in England, Scotland or Wales
- contact the Jobseeker's Allowance Processing Centre if you live in Northern Ireland.

You do not need to contact DWP unless it has been more than 14 days since you applied and you have not heard anything.

If you disagree with a decision
You can challenge a decision about your claim. This is called asking for mandatory reconsideration.

Documents you need to bring to your interview
You'll need to bring all of the following:
- one photographic proof of identity
- one proof of address
- one further proof of identity.

If you have a P45 from your employer, bring this to your interview. When you present it, tell your work coach if you've already received or claimed a tax refund from HMRC for the current tax year. You can also use your P45 as your further proof of identity.

Photographic proof of identity
Examples include your:

- current passport
- driving licence
- biometric residence permit
- certificate of naturalisation as a British citizen
- permanent residence permit.

Proof of address

Examples include a:
- payslip or pension statement dated within the last 6 months
- utility bill dated within the last 6 months
- Council Tax bill dated within the last 6 months
- student loan documentation.

Further proof of identity

Examples include your:
- P60
- savings account book
- personal cheque book
- current debit, credit or store card with a statement confirming the card details
- Utility bills can be used for proof of address and as further proof of identity if they are from different suppliers.

Support at your interview

You can take someone with you to your JSA interview.

Contact your Jobcentre Plus before the interview if you need:
- support because of a disability or health condition (for example, if you're deaf and need a sign language interpreter)
- a foreign language interpreter and do not have someone who can help with interpretation.

Sign an agreement to look for work ('Claimant Commitment')

At your JSA interview, you must sign an agreement about what steps you'll take to look for a job. This is called a 'Claimant Commitment'. You and your work coach will agree what goes in your Claimant Commitment. This could include:

- what you need to do to look for work - for example registering with recruitment agencies, writing a CV
- how many hours you need to spend looking for work each week
- What you agree to do will depend on things like:
- your health
- your responsibilities at home
- how much help you need to get work or increase your income.

After your JSA interview

The Department for Work and Pensions (DWP) will write to you to either:

- let you know you are eligible for JSA and how much you'll get
- explain why you're not eligible for JSA.

You will not need to do what you've agreed in your Claimant Commitment if you're not eligible for JSA.

Your JSA claim

When you apply to claim JSA, your work coach will make an agreement with you to look for work. This agreement is called a 'Claimant Commitment'. Your Claimant Commitment could include:

- what you need to do to look for work - for example registering with recruitment agencies or writing a CV
- how many hours you need to spend looking for work each week.

You should continue to do all the things you have agreed to do if you can do them safely. You can search and apply for work using the 'Find a job' service. You must tell Jobcentre Plus if your circumstances change, for example you start working or your income changes.

Attending regular appointments
Your work coach will arrange appointments with you every 1 to 2 weeks. At these appointments, you must show your work coach what you've been doing to look for work, for example proof of job applications and interviews. If you're a victim of domestic abuse you might be able to get a break of up to 13 weeks from job seeking - speak to your work coach if you need this support.

When payment can be reduced or stopped
Your JSA payments can be reduced or stopped for a period if you do not do something your work coach asks you to do. This is called being 'sanctioned'. For example, if you:
- do not take part in an appointment with your work coach
- do not accept or keep to your agreement to look for work
- turn down a job or training course
- do not apply for any jobs you're told about
- do not take part in any interviews you're invited to
- do not go to any training booked for you or take part in employment schemes.

You may also be sanctioned if you:

- are not available to start work straight away
- choose to take a pay cut at your current job without a good reason
- have your pay cut at your current job because of something you did, such as your behaviour
- leave your last job or training without good reason or because of your behaviour.

Contact Jobcentre Plus as soon as possible if any of these apply to you. You may be able to keep your payment if you have good reason. You'll be told how long your payment will be reduced or stopped for. It could be for up to 26 weeks (about 6 months).

If your JSA payment is reduced or stopped
If your payment is reduced or stopped, you should keep looking for work. Your benefit payment could be affected for longer if you do not. If you disagree with the decision to stop payment, you can ask for the decision to be looked at again - this is called 'mandatory reconsideration'. If you disagree with the outcome of the mandatory reconsideration, you can appeal to the Social Security and Child Support Tribunal. You should continue with any JSA claim until the dispute is settled.

If you claim Housing Benefit or Council Tax Reduction
You should contact your local council immediately. They'll tell you what to do to continue getting support.

If your claim is ended

If you get income based JSA, your claim may be ended if you're not available for or actively seeking work. You cannot apply for income based JSA again. Instead, check if you're eligible for Universal Credit and eligible for New Style Jobseeker's Allowance (JSA). You could get both at the same time.

Hardship payments

If you were claiming income based JSA, you may be able to get a hardship payment if your JSA payments have been stopped. You do not have to pay it back. A hardship payment is a reduced amount (usually 60%) of your JSA. If you were claiming New Style Jobseeker's Allowance (JSA), you cannot get a hardship payment.

Eligibility

You can get a hardship payment if you cannot pay for rent, heating, food or other basic needs for you or your child. You must be 18 or over. You'll have to show that you've tried to find the money from somewhere else, such as borrowing from a friend or working extra hours.

How to claim

Speak to your Jobcentre Plus adviser or work coach to find out how to claim a hardship payment.
Jobcentre Plus
Telephone: 0800 169 0310
Textphone: 0800 169 0314
Welsh language: 0800 328 1744
Monday to Friday, 8am to 6pm

If you're getting income based JSA

As long as you're still eligible, you'll keep getting income-based Jobseeker's Allowance (JSA) until your circumstances change. Jobcentre Plus will talk to you about your options. If you're eligible you might be able to claim Universal Credit. You need to take reasonable steps to look for work while getting JSA. You must tell Jobcentre Plus if your circumstances change, for example you start working or your income changes.

Working hours and income

If you start working more than 16 hours a week, you might stop being eligible for JSA. You might stop being eligible for income-based JSA if:

- your partner starts working 24 hours or more a week, or increases their hours to 16 hours or more a week
- your savings increase to £16,000 or more (including your partner's savings)
- You cannot apply for income-based JSA any more. Instead, check if you're eligible for Universal Credit and New Style JSA. You could get both at the same time.

Income support-Overview

You can no longer make a new claim for Income Support. If you're on a low income and need help to cover your living costs, you can apply for Universal Credit instead.

If you already get Income Support

You will continue to get Income Support if all of the following still apply to you (and your partner, if you have one):

- you have no income or a low income, and no more than £16,000 in savings
- you're not in full-time paid work (you can work less than 16 hours a week, and your partner can work less than 24 hours a week)
- you're between 16 and Pension Credit qualifying age
- you live in England, Scotland or Wales - there are different rules for Northern Ireland

You must also be at least one of the following:
- pregnant
- a lone parent (including a lone adoptive parent) with a child under 5
- a lone foster parent with a child under 16
- a single person looking after a child under 16 before they're adopted
- a carer
- on maternity, paternity or parental leave
- unable to work and you receive Statutory Sick Pay, Incapacity Benefit or Severe Disablement Allowance
- in full-time education (not university), aged between 16 and 20, and a parent
- in full-time education (not university), aged between 16 and 20, and not living with a parent or someone acting as a parent
- a refugee learning English - your course needs to be at least 15 hours a week, and you must have started it within 12 months of entering the UK
- in custody or due to attend court or a tribunal.

You do not need a permanent address - for example, you can continue to claim if you:

- sleep rough
- live in a hostel or care home.

You must continue to report any changes to your circumstances. You do not need to do anything else unless you are contacted by the Department for Work and Pensions (DWP).

If you're moving to Universal Credit

If your Income Support claim is ending because you're making a new claim for Universal Credit, you'll automatically continue to get the amount of Income Support you currently receive, as long as you're still eligible. You'll normally get this for 2 weeks, starting from the date of your new claim. DWP will write to you telling you how this works. You do not need to pay this money back, and it will not affect the amount of Universal Credit you get.

If you disagree with a decision

You can challenge a decision about your claim. This is called asking for mandatory reconsideration. Income Support includes:
- a basic payment (personal allowance)
- extra payments (premiums).

Your income and any savings (over £5,999) can affect how much you get.

Personal allowance (2024/5)

Your situation	Weekly payment
Single - age 16 to 24	£71.70

Your situation	Weekly payment
Single - age 25 or over	£90.50
Lone parent - age 16 to 17	£71.70
Lone parent - age 18 or over	£90.50
Couples - both under 18	£71.70
Couples - both under 18 getting 'higher rate'	£108.30
Couples - one under 18, the other 18 to 24	£71.70
Couples - one under 18, the other 25 or over	£90.50
Couples - one under 18, one over getting 'higher rate'	£142.25
Couples - both 18 or over	£142.25

Higher rate

The higher rate applies if either of you is responsible for a child, or if each of you would be eligible for one of the following if you were not a couple:

- Employment and Support Allowance
- Income Support
- Jobseeker's Allowance.

Premiums

An Income Support 'premium' is extra money based on your circumstances, for example if:

- your partner is a pensioner
- you're disabled or a carer.

The benefit cap

The benefit cap limits the total amount of benefit you can get. It applies to most people aged 16 or over who have not reached State Pension age. Some individual benefits are not affected, but it may affect the total amount of benefit you get.

Housing benefit

Housing Benefit can help you pay your rent if you're unemployed, on a low income or claiming benefits. It's being replaced by Universal Credit.

You can only make a new claim for Housing Benefit if either of the following apply:
- you have reached State Pension age
- you're in supported, sheltered or temporary housing.

You've reached State Pension age

If you're single you can make a new claim for Housing Benefit.

If you're over State Pension age and live with your partner

You can make a new claim for Housing Benefit if any of the following apply:
- you and your partner have both reached State Pension age
- one of you has reached State Pension age and started claiming Pension Credit (for you as a couple) before 15 May 2019
- you're in supported, sheltered or temporary housing.

If you're over State Pension age and have an existing claim

Your existing claim will not be affected if, before 15 May 2019, you:

- were getting Housing Benefit
- had reached State Pension age.

It does not matter if your partner is under State Pension age. If your circumstances change and your Housing Benefit is stopped, you cannot start getting it again unless you and your partner are eligible to make a new claim. You can apply for Universal Credit if you're not eligible.

If you're in supported, sheltered or temporary housing
You can make a new claim if:
- you're living in temporary accommodation, such as a B&B arranged by your council
- you're living in a refuge for survivors of domestic abuse
- you're living in sheltered or supported housing (such as a hostel) which provides you with 'care, support or supervision'.

If you do not get 'care, support or supervision' through your supported or sheltered housing, you can apply for Universal Credit to help with housing costs. If you're in supported, sheltered or temporary housing, you can apply for Universal Credit to help with other living costs.

When you may not be able to claim
Usually, you will not get Housing Benefit if:
- your savings are over £16,000 - unless you get Guarantee Credit of Pension Credit
- you're paying a mortgage on your own home - you may be able to get Support for Mortgage Interest (SMI)
- you live in the home of a close relative

- you're already claiming Universal Credit (unless you're in temporary or supported housing)
- you live with your partner and they are already claiming Housing Benefit
- you're a full-time student
- you're residing in the UK as a European Economic Area (EEA) jobseeker
- you're an asylum seeker or sponsored to be in the UK
- you're subject to immigration control and your granted leave states that you cannot claim public funds
- you're a Crown Tenant
- you've reached State Pension age but your live-in partner has not - unless you had an existing claim as a couple before 15 May 2019.

You may be able to get other help with housing costs. If not, you'll need to claim Universal Credit instead.

What you'll get

You may get help with all or part of your rent. There's no set amount of Housing Benefit and what you get will depend on whether you rent privately or from a council.

Council and social housing rent

How much you get depends on:
- your 'eligible' rent
- if you have a spare room
- your household income - including benefits, pensions and savings (over £6,000)

- your circumstances, for example the age of people in the house or if someone has a disability.

Eligible rent
Your eligible rent is the amount used to calculate your Housing Benefit claim. It's your actual rent plus any service charges you have to pay (such as for lift maintenance or a communal laundry) but not things like heating or water costs for your home.

Spare bedrooms
Your Housing Benefit could be reduced if you live in council or social housing and have a spare bedroom. The reduction is:
- 14% of the 'eligible rent' for 1 spare bedroom
- 25% of the 'eligible rent' for 2 or more spare bedrooms.

Example
Your eligible rent is £100 per week, but you have 1 spare bedroom. That means your eligible rent is reduced by 14%, to £86 per week. Your Housing Benefit will be calculated using that figure.

Sharing bedrooms
The following are expected to share:
- an adult couple
- 2 children under 16 of the same sex
- 2 children under 10 (regardless of sex)

The following can have their own bedroom:
- a single adult (16 or over)

- a child that would normally share but shared bedrooms are already taken, for example you have 3 children and 2 already share
- a couple or children who cannot share because of a disability or medical condition
- an overnight carer for you, your partner, your child or another adult - this is only if the carer does not live with you but sometimes has to stay overnight.

One spare bedroom is allowed for:
- an approved foster carer who is between placements but only for up to 52 weeks from the end of the last placement
- a newly approved foster carer for up to 52 weeks from the date of approval if no child is placed with them during that time.

Rooms used by students and members of the armed or reserve forces will not be counted as 'spare' if they're away and intend to return home.

Private rent

If you rent privately, your eligible rent amount is either your Local Housing Allowance (LHA) rate or your actual rent, whichever is lower. The LHA rate is based on:
- where you live
- your household size - find out how many bedrooms you're eligible for.

How much you can get

How much you get depends on:

- the lower figure of your 'eligible' rent or LHA rate
- your household income including benefits, pensions and savings (over £6,000)
- your circumstances (for example your age or whether you have a disability).

Contact your local council if you're living in:

- a houseboat or a mooring
- a caravan site
- a room with any meals included in the rent (sometimes known as a boarding home)
- a hostel
- a Rent Act protected property.

Exception

If you've been getting Housing Benefit since before 7 April 2008, these limits only apply if you:

- change address
- have a break in your claim for Housing Benefit.

How you're paid

The way you get paid Housing Benefit by your council depends on the type of tenant you are. If you're a:

- council tenant, it's paid into your rent account (you will not receive the money)
- private or housing association tenant, it's paid into your bank or building society account (rarely by cheque).

The benefit cap

The benefit cap limits the total amount of benefit you can get. It applies to most people aged 16 or over who have not reached State Pension age. If you're affected, your Housing Benefit will go down to make sure that the total amount of benefit you get is not more than the cap level. You'll need to provide some information and evidence to support your claim for Housing Benefit. You'll get Housing Benefit faster if you have this available when you make your claim. You'll need to know:

- how much rent you pay
- whether anything else is included in the rent, such as water, gas or electricity charges
- if you pay any service charges, including building maintenance or insurance
- your landlord or agent's details.

Special types of tenancy

If your current tenancy started in 1997 or earlier and you rent from a private landlord, you'll need to know if you have an 'assured tenancy'. You can check your tenancy on the Shelter website. If you live in and pay rent for a government property (a 'Crown Tenant'), you're not entitled to Housing Benefit. This includes armed forces living in service family accommodation (SFA).

Evidence you'll have to provide

You'll need to provide original documents, not copies. The supporting evidence you'll need includes:

- your most recent payslips (5 if paid weekly, or 2 if paid monthly)

- bank or building society statements for the last 2 full months
- proof of other income or investments, including shares, ISAs or Premium Bonds.
- proof of income for any non-dependants living with you, such as adult relatives or friends

You'll also need proof of your partner's name and address. You cannot use the same document to prove both their name and address. Provide any 2 of the following:
- UK photocard driving licence
- current passport
- birth or marriage certificate
- biometric residence permit
- certificate of registration or naturalisation
- permanent residence card
- letter from HMRC or the Home Office
- recent utility bill
- recent bank or building society statement
- recent benefit award statements.

If you rent from a private landlord

You'll also need to provide one of the following:
- a tenancy agreement or rent book
- a letter from your landlord confirming your tenancy - this is usually supplied at the start of your tenancy.

You can either apply:
- through your local council
- as part of a Pension Credit claim if you're eligible for this

You'll need to provide evidence to support your Housing Benefit claim.

If you're applying for Pension Credit

You can apply for Housing Benefit as part of your Pension Credit application. Apply for Pension Credit online or contact the Pension Service to claim. The Pension Service will send details of your claim for Housing Benefit to your council.

Pension Service
Telephone: 0800 99 1234
Textphone: 0800 169 0133
Relay UK (if you cannot hear or speak on the phone): 18001 then 0800 99 1234
Monday to Friday, 8am to 6pm

Claiming in advance and backdating

You can claim in advance by up to 13 weeks (or 17 weeks if you're aged 60 or over), for example if you're moving. You will not usually get any money before you move. You might also be able to get your claim backdated - ask your council.

Appeal a decision

If you're unhappy with a housing benefit decision, you can challenge the decision by:
- asking the council to review their decision
- appealing against it at a tribunal.

You can get free help and advice from:
- Citizens Advice or Shelter.

Council Tax Reduction-What is Council Tax Reduction?

Council Tax Reduction (also known as Council Tax Support) is a benefit to help people who are on a low income or claiming certain benefits to pay their Council Tax bill. You can make a claim whether you own your home or you're renting, and your employment status won't have an impact on your claim.

How much Council Tax Reduction will I get?

There's no set amount of Council Tax Reduction. What you get depends on your circumstances and where you live. Each local council operates its own Council Tax Reduction scheme, so the amounts of support given across the country may vary. Wherever you live, the amount of Council Tax Reduction you get depends on many factors, including:

- your age
- your income, including any benefits you receive
- your savings
- who you live with
- how much Council Tax you pay..

You may get more Council Tax Reduction if you receive a disability or carer's benefit.

If you receive the Guarantee Credit part of Pension Credit you may even get your Council Tax paid in full. If you don't get Guarantee Credit but have a low income and less than £16,000 in savings, you may still get some help. If you're not over State Pension age, the Council Tax Reduction you're entitled to is worked out using 'working age scheme' rules which tend to be less generous. Check these rules with your local council.

Am I eligible for Council Tax Reduction?
If you're on a low income or receiving certain benefits, you might be eligible for Council Tax Reduction.But whether you're eligible in your area, and what you might be eligible for, is up to your local council. Each council has their own rules so you should check what the rules are in your area.

The range of other help available if you are in urgent need
Emergency grants, loans and money help. There are options if you need help quickly for urgent things like:
- food
- rent or deposits
- gas and electric bills
- moving home or buying furniture,

You can sometimes get a grant or loan in an emergency or crisis situation. For example, if you lose your job or home and cannot meet your needs. Before you apply, check you are getting all the benefits you are entitled to.

How to find a grant
A grant does not have to be paid back so is better than a loan. You could try to get a grant through:
- a charity
- your council
- another hardship fund,

Help with money from your local council

Most councils can help with emergency expenses for food, bills, or emergency housing costs. Councils can:
- give money directly to residents
- offer vouchers instead of money
- fund local charities that help residents.

Councils have received extra money to help with the cost-of-living crisis. Get emergency money help from your local council
- Find your local council website on GOV.UK
- Search 'household support' or 'local welfare scheme' on your council's website
- Phone, email or visit their office in person if you cannot find any information online.

Councils have a separate scheme for people who cannot afford rent.

Council help to stop you losing your home

You can get help from the council if you're facing eviction or your home is unaffordable. The council could use money from its homeless prevention fund to help you stay in your home. For example, by clearing your arrears.

Other hardship funds

You can ask other organisations about hardship funds. For example, your:
- energy supplier
- trade union if you're a member
- university, college or student union.

Citizens Advice has more on grants to help with energy debts.

Other help you do not have to pay back
You can get extra financial help if you claim universal credit for things like rent, childcare and medical costs.

Discretionary housing payments
You can ask for a discretionary housing payment (DHP) if you cannot pay your full rent with your universal credit or housing benefit.

Free food from a food bank
Food banks provide at least 3 days of food for people with a food voucher. They are run by charities and community groups. Ask for a food voucher from a doctor, health visitor, social worker, school or advice service. Find a food bank on the Trussell Trust website.

Energy bills
If you cannot get a grant, you can still ask your supplier to:
- delay your bill
- remove late payment charges
- allow you to pay over a longer period.

You could also benefit from schemes to help pay energy bills like:
- cheaper tariffs for people with low income
- the warm home discount
- winter fuel payments.

Water
You can get help if you struggle to pay your water bills. You could also save money with a water meter if you have a larger home with

spare bedrooms. But it might cost more if you have a large family or live in a smaller home.

Broadband and mobile packages

You can often get cheaper internet and phone packages if you claim benefits like universal credit or pension credit. These lower tariffs do not always appear on comparison websites. End Furniture Poverty www.endfurniturepoverty.org has:
- advice on finding free furniture and white goods
- a local welfare assistance finder – search for your council scheme.

How to find a loan

Loans have to be paid back. A loan could help with an emergency expense but it:
- usually means you have less money each month until the loan is repaid
- can lead to longer term debt problems, especially if the interest rate is high
- Look for interest free loans. Make sure you can afford the repayments.

Interest free loans from the council

Councils may offer interest free loans if you have urgent needs. Local schemes set out:
- who can get help
- how much you can borrow
- when it must be paid back.

If you're facing eviction or homelessness the council might offer a loan to:
- pay off rent or mortgage arrears
- use as a deposit for another tenancy

Universal credit advances

You can ask for a universal credit advance during the 5-week wait for your first payment. You might need an advance if you cannot afford food, rent or important bills while you wait.

An advance is an interest free loan from the Department of Work and Pensions (DWP). You can pay it back over 2 years but your monthly universal credit payments will be lower while you pay back the advance.

Budgeting advances or loans from the DWP

You can also apply for a:
- budgeting advance if you get universal credit
- budgeting loan if you get certain other benefits.

You must have been getting universal credit or another low-income benefit for at least 6 months to get a budgeting advance or loan. A budgeting advance or loan can be used for:
- household items such as cookers, fridges or beds
- rent in advance or removal costs if moving home
- repairs or security improvements to your home.

Credit union loans

You need to be a member of a credit union to apply for a loan. Credit union loans are usually more expensive than personal loans from a bank or building society but it may be easier to get a loan if you have a poor credit history. Credit union loans are not interest free.

Avoid payday loans and doorstep lenders
These types of loans are expensive and often make your financial situation worse. StepChange debt charity has advice on:
- payday loans and dealing with debt
- doorstep lending and illegal loan sharks.

****